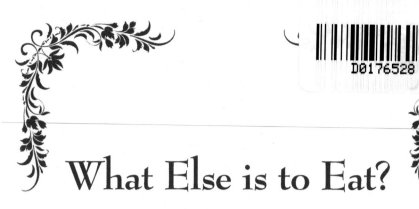

What Else is to Eat?

The Dairy-, Egg-, and Nut-Free Food Allergy Cookbook

Linda Marienhoff Coss

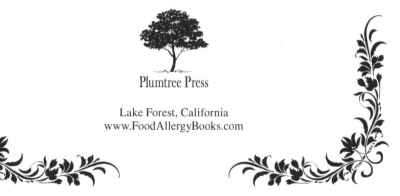

Plumtree Press

Lake Forest, California
www.FoodAllergyBooks.com

WHAT ELSE IS TO EAT?
THE DAIRY-, EGG-, AND NUT-FREE
FOOD ALLERGY COOKBOOK

Plumtree Press/September, 2008

All rights reserved.

Copyright © 2008 by Linda Marienhoff Coss

Cover and Interior Production by 1106 Design

Interior Page Border Art Design by Kevin Coss

Permission should be addressed in writing to:
LindaCoss@FoodAllergyBooks.com or
Plumtree Press, P.O. Box 1313, Lake Forest, California 92609-1313

Library of Congress Control Number: 2008923963

ISBN 978-0-9702785-2-4

Printed in the United States of America

Dedication

I dedicate this book to my children,
Jason and Kevin,
who have grown up into
such fine young men,
and to you,
the reader,
who has allowed me
into your kitchen
and your life.

Also by Linda Coss

What's to Eat?
The Milk-Free, Egg-Free, Nut-Free Food Allergy Cookbook

How To Manage Your Child's Life-Threatening Food Allergies
Practical Tips For Everyday Life

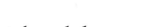

Acknowledgements

I would like to thank my children, Jason and Kevin, for their patience with all of my kitchen experimentation (when you look back on your childhood you'll always remember the "4-star recipe rating system"); my parents, for everything; Scott Greenberg, for all of his love, support, and encouragement; all of my recipe testers, including Jennifer Bingham, Alisa Fleming, Scott Greenberg, Diana Marienhoff, and more; Ruth Greenberg and Diana Marienhoff for their editing assistance; and all of the people who purchased my first cookbook and encouraged me to write a second.

Warning and Disclaimer

The information contained in this book is not intended to replace the advice of your physician, nor is it meant to replace medical diagnosis or treatment. If you have or suspect that you have food allergies, you are strongly urged to seek out appropriate medical advice. If you are already under the care of a physician for your food allergies, be sure to discuss with him or her any changes that you intend to make in your diet.

If you or someone that you are cooking for suffers from severe food allergies, it is imperative that you check the ingredient statement of each item that you use in your cooking in order to ensure that the item does not contain any food allergens. This must be done every time that the item is purchased, as food manufacturers often change their ingredients without notice. In addition, you must be sure that any open containers of food to be used in your cooking have not been "contaminated" with a food allergen. For example, a jar of jelly which does not have any dairy, egg, or nut ingredients listed in its ingredient panel will contain peanut if at some point in time a knife that had peanut butter on it had been placed in the jelly jar; in this case, the jelly should not be eaten by a person who has peanut allergy.

No promises or warranties, express or implied, as to the appropriateness of any food or recipe for a particular person's diet is made by this book. No liability will be assumed by anyone affiliated with the writing, production, or distribution of this book for any damages arising from the preparation or consumption of the foods described herein, whether such losses are special, incidental, consequential, or otherwise.

The reader accepts sole responsibility for the use of the information contained in this book.

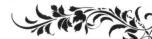

Table of Contents

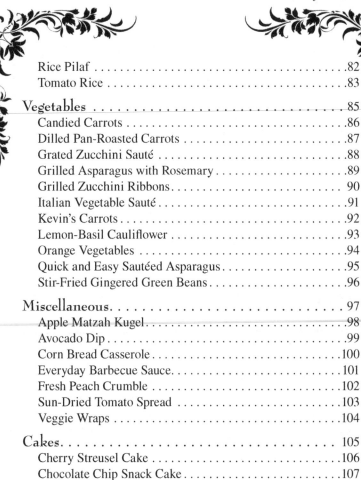

Introduction

It's been 16 years since I began my food allergy journey, and a lot has changed since then. When I first started on this road it was a very lonely and uncrowded place. Few people (including, it seemed, most medical professionals) had heard of life-threatening food allergies, and everyone thought I had gone off the deep end when I explained the sorts of precautions I had to take to keep my son safe.

Almost no resources were available, the internet didn't exist (or if it did no one in the general public had heard of it), food manufacturers weren't required to include ingredient panels on their packaging at all, and the Americans with Disabilities Act was so new that it was not yet widely enforced. With no maps to guide the way, the food allergy road was a very difficult road to travel.

Well, that sleepy little food allergy road has now become a traffic-choked food allergy highway. Although it is still a very difficult road to travel, there are now maps, guidebooks, news reports, and lots of fellow travelers with whom to share the journey. In fact, so many children now have life-threatening food allergies that the topic is regularly in the news, food labeling laws have been passed specifically to help the food-allergic, and school districts across the country have been forced by necessity to create policies to cope with the issue.

My own life, of course, has changed as well. As I write this, my food-allergic son is awaiting his college acceptance letters. It fact, it was the realization that he would soon be moving out of the house (and that I, theoretically, could dust off my long-forgotten recipes for quiche and cashew chicken) that motivated me to finally finish this book!

As you may know, *What Else is to Eat?* is the sequel to my first cookbook, *What's to Eat?* To be honest, when I put the finishing

touches on that book I told my friends that I was through creating recipes and I was never doing this again. Ha! Ha! Never say never! I gave it up for a while…I poured my energy into writing and self-publishing another book, *How To Manage Your Child's Life-Threatening Food Allergies: Practical Tips For Everyday Life*…and then I started experimenting in the kitchen once again.

When I created the recipes for *What's to Eat?* I was a stay-at-home mom with two little boys. Now I'm a working mom (yes, I do have a "day job" – I'm a freelance marketing copywriter) with two teenage boys. My life has become much more hectic, and like many people, the time that I have available to devote to cooking has shrunk. If you have both of my cookbooks, you probably won't mind that this one has an even greater emphasis on "fast and easy," especially in the dinner department.

To those of you who may object to the fact that not all of my recipes (in either of my cookbooks) are "toddler friendly," I'll apologize now. The reality is that not all food allergy sufferers are small children, and there is a big need for delicious hypo-allergenic recipes that are suitable for a variety of diners and occasions. Besides, even those with small children often choose to make their entire home allergen-free and sometimes need ideas for what to serve at more adult-oriented events!

So here for your enjoyment is a whole collection of kitchen-tested recipes for wonderful food that happens to be dairy-, egg-, and nut-free. Whether you're just starting off on your food allergy journey or a seasoned traveler, I sincerely hope that this collection of recipes helps make coping with food allergies just a little bit easier for you.

Bon appétit!

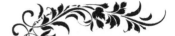
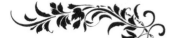

Food Allergy Cooking

Whether you are new to the food allergy world or a "seasoned pro," welcome! This book contains 115 kitchen-tested recipes, all of which are completely free of milk, egg, peanut and tree nut ingredients.

In the world of food allergy cooking, having a collection of appropriate recipes is just the first step. Unlike cooking for most people, cooking for a person who has severe food allergies requires that you take a number of precautions. Because food allergies can be life-threatening, following appropriate food safety protocols can mean the difference between an enjoyable meal and an ambulance ride to the emergency room. To help you avoid allergic reactions, the information in this section is meant to acquaint you with the basics of food allergy cooking.

Check the Ingredient Statement

When purchasing food for a person who has severe food allergies, every item (including those that will be used as ingredients in recipes) must be scrutinized to determine if it contains – or might be "contaminated" with – the forbidden allergens. *It is imperative that you check the ingredient panel of each item that you purchase, each time you purchase the product.* Avoid foods that contain the allergens you are avoiding. Be aware that ingredients can and do change without warning.

In the U.S., the Food Allergy Labeling and Consumer Protection Act (FALCPA) affects all foods regulated by the FDA that are required to have ingredient statements. FALCPA requires that if a food contains milk, egg, peanut, tree nut, wheat, soybean, fish, or shellfish this must be stated in plain English either in the ingredient statement or in a "contains" statement immediately after or adjacent to the ingredient statement. However, as of this writing foods regulated by the USDA (such as meats and poultry) or the Alcohol, Tobacco Tax and Trade Bureau (such as alcoholic beverages) are not covered by this law.

Watch out for Cross-Contamination at the Manufacturing Facility

Those who are extremely sensitive must also watch out for the "cross-contamination" that can occur when food manufacturers make a variety of products on the same production line. For example, a company may produce semi-sweet chocolate chips on the same machinery as milk chocolate chips, with the result being that the semi-sweet chips may contain traces of milk.

Although some companies will put "may contain" or "produced on the same equipment as" warnings on these products, as of this writing U.S. laws do not require food manufacturers to warn consumers of possible cross-contamination. Therefore, the absence of a "may contain traces of X" notice does not necessarily mean that the food does not contain traces of X. The only way to be certain that a particular food is not produced on the same machinery or in the same facility as an allergen-containing product is to contact the food's manufacturer and ask.

Avoid Cross-Contamination in Your Kitchen

Foods can also become "contaminated" with off-limits ingredients while they are in your home. For example, if you place a knife that has peanut butter on it into a jar of jelly, that jelly would now contain peanut, and should not be consumed by a person who has peanut allergy.

Take steps to avoid contaminating otherwise "safe" foods during the cooking or serving process. Do not use the same utensils to simultaneously prepare allergenic and non-allergenic dishes. Wash your hands before cooking, and be sure to use clean cutting boards, knives, mixing bowls, utensils, baking pans, etc., in the preparation of non-allergenic foods.

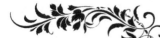

My "Ingredient-Listing Protocol"

Throughout this book I have placed all packaged ingredients that are not "pure" products (such as pure cane sugar, which by definition should only contain sugar) in **bold** as a reminder for you to double-check the ingredient panels of these products. In cases where I know that some varieties of that item commonly contain dairy, egg, or nut ingredients, I have specified "dairy-free," "egg-free," or whatever.

For example, because most margarines contain milk or milk derivatives, all recipes in this book that require margarine specify "dairy-free **margarine**." This does not mean that you should not also check the ingredient panel of your margarine for eggs and nuts. This means that, as of the time of this writing, I personally have never seen eggs or nuts listed as ingredients in margarine – although I have seen dairy products listed as margarine ingredients.

I have also listed ingredients in bold if I think there's a good chance the item might be cross-contaminated with an allergen. An example of this is raisins. Although to the best of my knowledge as of this writing all of the major brands of raisins are safe, I also know that dried fruits sold at roadside stands and specialty stores are often processed on the same machinery as nuts.

Remember, it is always your responsibility to ensure that every ingredient you use is completely dairy-, egg-, and nut-free.

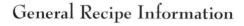

General Recipe Information

General Information

Preparation times are approximate, and assume that all ingredients and equipment needed have been assembled prior to beginning the recipe preparation.

Cooking times are approximate, due to variations in ovens, oven temperatures, and altitude.

Preheating oven: Always preheat your oven to the specified temperature before placing the dish in the oven. Although heating times will vary, most ovens will heat to the designated temperature in about ten minutes.

"Salt and pepper to taste" means that you should add the amount of salt and pepper that you prefer. Because personal preferences for salt and pepper vary widely, in many recipes I left it to your discretion to determine how much of these seasonings to add.

How to Measure Ingredients

Liquid ingredients: Place liquid measuring cup on level surface, pour in ingredient, and read markings on cup at eye level.

Dry ingredients: Spoon ingredient loosely into an appropriate-sized dry measuring cup or measuring spoon, piling high; level off with a metal spatula or straight-sided knife.

Brown sugar: Using the back of a spoon, pack brown sugar firmly into an appropriate-sized dry measuring cup until even with the rim of the measuring cup. When inverted out of the measuring cup, brown sugar should hold its shape. Brown sugar measured in this way is called "firmly packed."

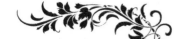

Shortening: Using a rubber spatula, pack shortening into an appropriate-sized dry measuring cup. Run spatula through shortening to release air; pack again and then level off.

Standard Baking Ingredients

All-purpose flour refers to standard (white) wheat flour; this is used in all recipes in this book that call for flour, unless whole wheat flour is specified. None of the recipes in this book call for cake flour.

Brown sugar is 100% pure cane brown sugar.

Chocolate chips are dairy- and nut-free semi-sweet chocolate chips. Please be aware that most brands of semi-sweet chocolate chips available in the supermarket are made on the same machinery as products that contain either dairy or nuts. For a current list of online sources for "safe" chocolate chips, please visit the resources page of my website at *www.FoodAllergyBooks.com*.

Cocoa is unsweetened 100% pure cocoa powder.

Egg substitute: The oil/water/baking powder mixture specified in most of the baked goods recipes in this book is an egg substitute. These ingredients must be mixed together in a separate bowl or cup until the mixture "fizzes" and the baking powder dissolves, and then added to the recipe as directed. For best results you should complete the recipe immediately after mixing the oil/water/baking powder mixture; do not set the unfinished batter aside until later in the day.

Margarine is dairy-free margarine, and is not "whipped" margarine. Try to find one with a high fat content, a low water content, and a "buttery" taste. A margarine that has a high water content will produce inferior baked goods. A good margarine can make a big difference in many of these recipes; if you are not satisfied with the performance of your margarine, try to find another acceptable brand.

Powdered sugar is also known as "confectioner's sugar."

Shortening is 100% vegetable shortening; do not use the "butter-flavored" varieties, as these may contain milk.

Sugar is 100% pure cane granulated sugar unless brown sugar or powdered sugar is specified.

Vegetable oil is 100% soybean oil.

White distilled vinegar is sold in bottles labeled as such, and should not be confused with white wine vinegar.

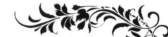

Recommended Equipment

If you're new to the world of food allergy cooking you may find yourself doing quite a bit more cooking than you did in the past, possibly working in a kitchen that's lacking some basic cooking and baking equipment.

To help you determine what equipment you need and what you can live without, here is a list of equipment needed to prepare the recipes contained in this book.

Pots, Pans, and Bakeware

2-quart saucepan
3-quart pot
4-quart pot
8-quart pot – optional, only used for 1 recipe in this book
12-inch skillet or sauté pan, preferably non-stick, with lid
9-inch by 13-inch glass or ceramic baking dish
large roasting pan – optional, only used for 1 recipe in this book
two 9-inch round cake pans
8-inch square cake pan
9-inch by 5-inch loaf pan
muffin pans – enough so you can make 12 standard-sized muffins
    at once (note: "standard" muffin pans hold about ⅓ cup batter
    per muffin)
cookie sheets, preferably rimmed
wire racks
Bundt pan – optional, only used for 1 recipe in this book
quiche pan – optional, only used for 1 recipe in this book

Measuring Equipment

measuring cups for measuring liquid ingredients
measuring cups for measuring dry ingredients
measuring spoons – used for both liquid and dry ingredients

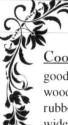

Cooking Utensils

good set of kitchen knives
wooden spoon
rubber or flexible silicone spatula
wide spatula – sometimes called a "pancake turner"
metal spatula – narrow-blade spatula used to spread frosting
   on cakes
slotted spoon
wire whisk
pastry blender
ladle
vegetable peeler
pastry brush
rolling pin – optional, only used for 1 recipe in this book
meat thermometer – optional, only used for 1 recipe in this book
heart-shaped cookie cutter – optional, only used for 1 recipe in
   this book

Miscellaneous Equipment

mixing bowls, preferably microwave-safe
cutting board
kitchen timer
thin mesh wire strainer – used for sifting dry ingredients for
   baked goods
colander
can opener
wire splatter guard – optional, only used for 1 recipe in this book
cookie press – optional, only used for 1 recipe in this book
Five 10-inch-long metal skewers – optional, only used for
   1 recipe in this book

Appliances

microwave oven
electric mixer – either hand-held or free-standing model –
   specified in 7 recipes in this book (but could also be used
   in many others)

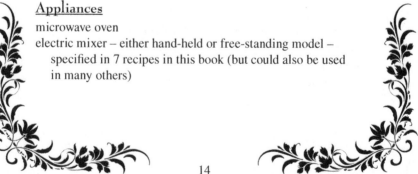

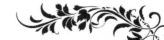

wok – used in 5 recipes in this book
5-quart slow cooker – used in 5 recipes in this book
food processor – used in 10 recipes in this book, most of which
  could also be made using a good blender plus possibly a hand-
  held grater, and a sharp knife
barbecue – the 9 grilling recipes in this book were all tested using
  a gas barbecue; none were tested with a charcoal barbecue

Notes

Soups
&
Salads

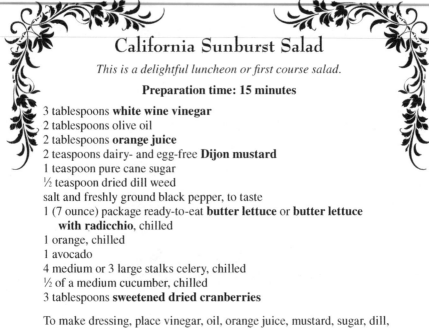

California Sunburst Salad

This is a delightful luncheon or first course salad.

Preparation time: 15 minutes

3 tablespoons **white wine vinegar**
2 tablespoons olive oil
2 tablespoons **orange juice**
2 teaspoons dairy- and egg-free **Dijon mustard**
1 teaspoon pure cane sugar
½ teaspoon dried dill weed
salt and freshly ground black pepper, to taste
1 (7 ounce) package ready-to-eat **butter lettuce** or **butter lettuce with radicchio**, chilled
1 orange, chilled
1 avocado
4 medium or 3 large stalks celery, chilled
½ of a medium cucumber, chilled
3 tablespoons **sweetened dried cranberries**

To make dressing, place vinegar, oil, orange juice, mustard, sugar, dill, salt, and pepper in a small bowl; mix well with a fork or small wire whisk. Set aside.

Tear lettuce into bite-size pieces. Peel orange, divide into sections, and cut each section into ¼-inch pieces. Peel, pit, and slice avocado. Thinly slice celery. Peel cucumber, cut in half lengthwise, and then slice thinly. Place prepared lettuce, orange, avocado, celery, and cucumber in a large salad bowl. Add cranberries and dressing; toss gently. Serve.

Makes 2 to 3 main-dish or 4 to 5 side-dish servings.

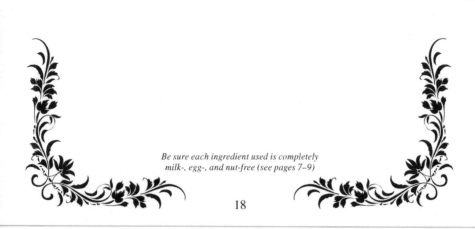

*Be sure each ingredient used is completely
milk-, egg-, and nut-free (see pages 7–9)*

Corn and Potato Soup

This makes a satisfying, chowder-like soup.

Preparation time: 15 minutes
Cooking time: 20 minutes

1 pound white rose potatoes (about 2 medium)
½ of a medium brown onion
3 medium stalks celery
1 tablespoon dairy-free **margarine**
1 teaspoon bottled **minced garlic**
1 (15 ounce) can **cream-style corn**
1 (14.5 ounce) can dairy- and egg-free **fat-free reduced-sodium
    chicken broth** (1¾ cups broth)
½ teaspoon ground nutmeg
salt and pepper to taste

Peel potatoes; dice into ¼-inch cubes. Set aside.

Peel and chop onion. Chop celery. Melt margarine in a 4-quart pot over medium-high heat. Add chopped onion, celery, and garlic; sauté about four minutes, until soft.

Stir in remaining ingredients, including diced potatoes. Cover and bring to a boil over high heat. Stir. Reduce heat to low and simmer, covered, for 20 minutes, stirring occasionally. Serve hot.

Makes 4 servings (1¼ cups each).

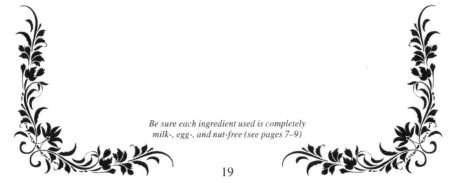

*Be sure each ingredient used is completely
milk-, egg-, and nut-free (see pages 7–9)*

Critics' Choice Chicken Salad

Company coming for lunch? Serve this terrific restaurant-style main dish salad and then sit back and enjoy the compliments.

Preparation and cooking time: 20 minutes

2 tablespoons **yellow cornmeal**
½ teaspoon dried rosemary, crumbled
¼ teaspoon paprika
½ pound thin-sliced chicken breast filets
1 tablespoon dairy-free **margarine**
1 medium Granny Smith apple, chilled
3 tablespoons canola or **vegetable oil**
2 tablespoons freshly squeezed lemon juice
2 tablespoons honey
1 tablespoon **raspberry vinegar** or **apple cider vinegar**
1 teaspoon poppy seeds
1 (10 ounce) bag washed and cut **romaine lettuce**, chilled
1 (11 ounce) can **mandarin oranges** packed in light syrup,
     chilled, drained
¼ cup **sweetened dried cranberries**

Place cornmeal, rosemary, and paprika in a large sealable plastic bag; seal and shake to mix. Rinse chicken (do not dry) and place in the bag with the cornmeal mixture. Seal the bag and shake to coat chicken with cornmeal mixture. Heat 1 tablespoon margarine in a 12-inch skillet over medium-high heat. Place coated chicken pieces in a single layer in skillet. Cook about 4 minutes per side, until juices run clear when chicken is pierced with a fork. Remove chicken from skillet and let cool 3 minutes.

While chicken is cooking, peel, core, and thinly slice apple; set aside. To make dressing place oil, lemon juice, honey, vinegar, and poppy seeds in a small bowl; mix well and set aside.

Slice the cooked and cooled chicken. Place lettuce in a large salad bowl. Arrange sliced apple, mandarin orange pieces, dried cranberries, and cooked and sliced chicken over lettuce. Pour prepared dressing over salad. Serve.

Makes 2 main-dish servings.

*Be sure each ingredient used is completely
milk-, egg-, and nut-free (see pages 7–9)*

Medley Soup

*My son Jason – who isn't usually a big fan of soup –
enjoyed this one so much that I let him name it! This
makes a hearty soup that is a meal in itself.*

Preparation and cooking time: 20 minutes

3 (5.5 ounce) cans **low-sodium 100% vegetable juice** (2 cups)
1 (14.5 ounce) can dairy- and egg-free **fat-free reduced-sodium
  chicken broth** (1¼ cups broth)
1 (14.5 ounce) can **diced and peeled tomatoes in tomato juice**,
  not drained
1 (8.5 ounce) can "no salt added" **whole kernel corn**, not drained
¼ cup chopped brown onion
½ cup peeled baby-cut carrots
½ tablespoon firmly packed fresh parsley leaves
½ cup dairy-, egg-, and nut-free **orzo pasta**
½ pound extra lean ground beef
1 teaspoon bottled **minced garlic**
½ teaspoon **seasoned salt**

Place vegetable juice, chicken broth, tomatoes (with juice), and corn
(with liquid) in a 4-quart pot. Cover and bring to a boil over high heat.

Peel and chop onion; set aside. Slice carrots into ⅛-inch-thick rounds.
Chop parsley.

When the soup comes to a boil, add sliced carrots, parsley, and orzo.
Return to boil over high heat, and then reduce heat to low and simmer,
covered, for 10 minutes.

Meanwhile, place ground beef, chopped onion, garlic, and seasoned salt
in a 10- or 12-inch skillet. Cook over medium-high heat until no pink
remains in meat, stirring frequently to break meat into small pieces.
Drain and discard fat. Add cooked meat mixture to cooked soup; stir.
Serve hot.

Makes 6 servings (1⅓ cups each).

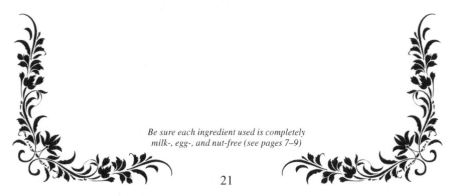

*Be sure each ingredient used is completely
milk-, egg-, and nut-free (see pages 7–9)*

Orange County Salmon Salad

*The sweet dressing in this main course salad is a perfect
accompaniment for the seasoned broiled salmon.*

Preparation and cooking time: 25 to 30 minutes

1 tablespoon firmly packed pure cane dark brown sugar
1 teaspoon ground mustard powder
1 teaspoon **mild curry powder**
½ teaspoon **lemon pepper**
¾ pound boneless, skinless salmon filet
1 (5 ounce) bag pre-washed **mixed baby greens**, chilled
1 ripe avocado
1 cup cherry tomatoes, chilled
2 tablespoons **orange juice**
1 tablespoon **balsamic vinegar**
1 tablespoon canola or **vegetable oil**
¼ teaspoon pure cane sugar
¼ teaspoon bottled **minced ginger**

Preheat broiler. Spray broiler pan with dairy-free **non-stick cooking
spray.**

Place brown sugar, ground mustard, curry powder, and lemon pepper
in a small bowl; mix well. Rinse salmon and pat dry with paper towels.
Press the seasoning mixture evenly onto both sides of salmon and then
place salmon on prepared broiler pan. Broil for about 7 to 8 minutes per
side, until cooked through.

While salmon is cooking, prepare salad. Place greens in a large salad
bowl. Peel and pit avocado, and then cut into cubes. Slice each tomato
in quarters. Arrange avocado and tomato over greens in bowl. To make
dressing, place remaining ingredients in a small bowl or measuring
cup; mix well.

Cut cooked salmon into bite-size pieces; arrange over salad in bowl.
Add salad dressing and toss. Serve immediately.

Makes 2 main-dish servings.

*Be sure each ingredient used is completely
milk-, egg-, and nut-free (see pages 7–9)*

Ready-in-a-Flash Picnic Salad

This recipe makes a large quantity of salad, perfect for serving as a side dish at a party.

Preparation time: 5 minutes
Marinating time: 10 minutes or more

¼ cup **ketchup**
¼ cup **red wine vinegar**
¼ cup canola oil
2 tablespoons honey
salt and pepper to taste (optional)
1 (12 ounce) bag **broccoli slaw**, chilled
1 (8 ounce) bag **shredded carrots**, chilled
1 cup **raisins**

To make dressing place ketchup, vinegar, oil, honey, and (optional) salt and pepper in a small bowl; mix well with a fork or wire whisk.

Place broccoli slaw, carrots, raisins, and dressing in a large serving bowl. Mix well. Refrigerate at least 10 minutes before serving.

Makes 9 servings (about ¾ cup each).

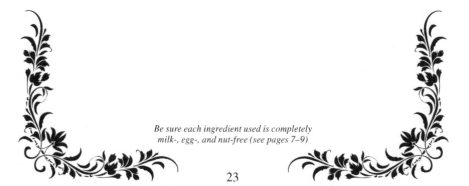

Be sure each ingredient used is completely milk-, egg-, and nut-free (see pages 7–9)

Seven Minute Soup

*Here's a great recipe for when you truly don't have time
to cook. Pair this with a nice dairy-, egg-, and nut-free
French bread and a light supper will be ready before the
kids finish washing their hands and setting the table!*

Preparation and cooking time: 7 minutes

2 (14.5 ounce) cans dairy- and egg-free **fat-free reduced-sodium
  chicken broth** (3½ cups broth)
1 (14.5 ounce) can **diced and peeled tomatoes in tomato juice,**
  not drained
1 (6 or 8 ounce) package fresh sliced button mushrooms
2 teaspoons **Italian seasoning**

Place chicken broth in a 3-quart pot. Cover and bring to a boil over
high heat.

While broth is boiling, heat a 12-inch skillet over medium-high heat.
Add tomatoes (with juice) and mushrooms. Sauté for four minutes,
stirring frequently.

Add sautéed vegetables and Italian seasoning to boiling chicken broth;
stir. Serve hot.

Makes 4 servings (1½ cups each).

*Be sure each ingredient used is completely
milk-, egg-, and nut-free (see pages 7–9)*

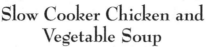

Slow Cooker Chicken and Vegetable Soup

There's nothing like a bowl of soup on a cold winter day.
Here's a satisfying version of that old favorite – chicken and
vegetable – for your slow cooker. If you prefer more of a stew
consistency, you can eliminate 1 can of chicken broth.

Preparation time: 20 minutes
Cooking time: 8 hours

1 large russet potato (about 14 to 16 ounces)
1 medium brown onion
1 stalk celery
¾ cup peeled baby-cut carrots
1 pound boneless, skinless chicken thighs
1 (14.5 ounce) can **diced and peeled tomatoes in tomato juice**,
    not drained
1 (8.5 ounce) can "no salt added" **whole kernel corn**
2 (14.5 ounce) cans dairy- and egg-free **fat-free reduced-sodium**
    chicken broth (3½ cups broth)
2 tablespoons dairy- and egg-free **Dijon mustard**
1 teaspoon paprika
½ teaspoon garlic salt
½ teaspoon ground sage
½ teaspoon pepper

Peel potato and chop into small pieces. Peel and chop onion. Thinly
slice celery. Slice carrots into thin rounds. Place prepared potato, onion,
celery, and carrots into a 5-quart slow cooker.

Trim fat off of chicken and then cut chicken into approximately 1-inch
pieces; place on top of vegetables in slow cooker. Pour canned tomatoes
and corn, with their liquids, on top of chicken.

Pour about 1 cup of chicken broth into a small bowl or measuring cup.
Add mustard, paprika, garlic salt, sage, and pepper; mix well. Add this
seasoned broth, as well as the remaining broth, to the slow cooker. Cover
and cook on low heat setting for 8 hours.

Makes 7 servings (about 1⅓ cups each).

Be sure each ingredient used is completely
milk-, egg-, and nut-free (see pages 7–9)

Spaghetti and Meatball Soup

*Okay, I'll admit it – this doesn't actually call for spaghetti,
because when I tested the recipe with spaghetti noodles
the pasta kept falling off the spoon. But "spiral pasta
and meatball soup" just didn't sound as good!*

Preparation time: 20 minutes
Cooking time: 10 minutes

2 (14.5 ounce) cans dairy- and egg-free **fat-free reduced-sodium chicken broth** (3½ cups broth)
1 (8 ounce) can **tomato sauce**
½ teaspoon dried oregano leaves
½ teaspoon dried basil leaves
½ teaspoon dried sage leaves
½ teaspoon dried thyme leaves
½ teaspoon pepper
¼ of a small brown onion
3 large cloves fresh garlic
½ pound extra lean ground beef or ground turkey
½ teaspoon dried parsley leaves
½ teaspoon **seasoned salt**
1 tablespoon olive oil
1 (8 ounce) package dairy-, egg-, and nut-free **spiral pasta**

Place chicken broth, tomato sauce, oregano, basil, sage, thyme, and pepper in a 4-quart pot; mix well. Cover and bring to a boil over high heat. Reduce heat to low and simmer, covered.

Peel and chop onion; you should have ¼ cup. Peel garlic and press through garlic press. Set aside.

Place ground meat, parsley, and seasoned salt in a medium mixing bowl; mix well. Form mixture into ½-inch-diameter mini meatballs. Heat olive oil in a 12-inch skillet over medium-high heat. Add meatballs and cook, occasionally stirring gently, until browned on all sides, about 2 to 3 minutes. Using a slotted spoon, remove meatballs from skillet and add to simmering soup. Add prepared onion and garlic to skillet and sauté over medium-high heat, stirring constantly, until onions are soft, about 2 minutes. Using a slotted spoon, remove onions and garlic from skillet and add to soup. Add pasta to soup. Cover and simmer over low heat for 10 minutes or until pasta is cooked, stirring once or twice during cooking time. Serve hot.

Makes 4 servings (about 1⅓ cups each).

*Be sure each ingredient used is completely
milk-, egg-, and nut-free (see pages 7–9)*

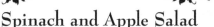

Spinach and Apple Salad

*This healthy and tasty side-dish salad makes a nice
accompaniment for a meat or chicken entrée.*

Preparation time: 10 to 12 minutes

2 tablespoons olive oil
2 tablespoons **white wine vinegar**
1 teaspoon pure cane sugar
1 teaspoon ground mustard powder
1 teaspoon dried basil leaves
salt and pepper to taste
2 small red apples, chilled
1 (6 ounce) bag pre-washed **baby spinach**, chilled
¼ cup **sweetened dried cranberries**
¼ cup minced fresh chives

To make dressing place oil, vinegar, sugar, mustard powder, basil,
salt, and pepper in a small bowl; mix well with a wire whisk or fork.
Set aside.

Peel and core apples. Cut each apple in half, and then cut each half into
thin slices.

To assemble salad, place spinach in a large salad bowl. Arrange apple
slices over spinach and then sprinkle cranberries and chives over
apples. Drizzle with dressing. Serve immediately.

Makes 4 servings (2 cups each).

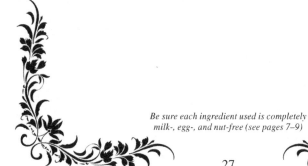

*Be sure each ingredient used is completely
milk-, egg-, and nut-free (see pages 7–9)*

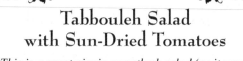

Tabbouleh Salad
with Sun-Dried Tomatoes

*This is a great picnic or potluck salad (as it won't
spoil the moment the sun comes out) or a nice
change-of-pace side dish to serve with dinner.*

Preparation and cooking time: 18 to 20 minutes

⅓ cup **sun-dried tomato halves** (the dry variety, not oil-packed)
1 (14.5 ounce) can dairy- and egg-free **fat-free reduced-sodium
  chicken broth** (1¼ cups broth)
1 cup bulgur (i.e., cracked wheat), uncooked
2 green onions (scallions)
¼ cup firmly packed fresh parsley leaves
1 medium clove fresh garlic
3 tablespoons freshly squeezed lemon juice
1 tablespoon olive oil
lemon slices or fresh parsley sprigs for garnish (optional)

Cut each sun-dried tomato half into 4 pieces. Place broth, bulgur, and
sun-dried tomatoes in a 3-quart pot; stir. Cover and bring to a boil over
high heat. Reduce heat to low and simmer, covered, for 10 minutes or
until bulgur is tender and liquid is absorbed.

While bulgur cooks, prepare rest of ingredients. Chop green onions,
including the green tops. Mince parsley. Set prepared onions and
parsley aside. Peel garlic and press through garlic press. To make
dressing place pressed garlic, lemon juice, and oil in a small mixing
bowl; mix well.

Place cooked bulgur mixture, chopped onions, minced parsley, and
dressing in a large serving bowl; mix well. If desired, garnish with
lemon slices or parsley sprigs. Either serve immediately or refrigerate
and serve chilled.

Makes 4 servings (¾ cup each).

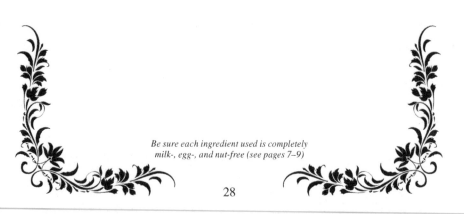

*Be sure each ingredient used is completely
milk-, egg-, and nut-free (see pages 7–9)*

Beef

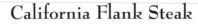

California Flank Steak

Here's an easy recipe for a delicious and flavorful steak. Pair this with some grilled vegetables for a great summer dinner.

Preparation time: 5 minutes
Marinating time: 24 hours
Cooking time: 20 minutes

1 (5.5 ounce) can **low-sodium 100% vegetable juice** (about ⅔ cup)
¼ cup dairy-free **low-sodium soy sauce**
¼ cup firmly packed pure cane dark brown sugar
2 tablespoons **Worcestershire sauce**
1 teaspoon bottled **minced garlic**
1 tablespoon dried rosemary, crumbled
1 tablespoon dried basil leaves
1 flank steak, about 1½ pounds

To make marinade, place all ingredients except steak in a medium bowl; mix well. Trim all fat from steak and then place steak and marinade in a large sealable plastic bag. Seal bag and refrigerate for 24 hours, turning the bag over once about halfway through the marinating time.

Heat gas grill to high. Grill steak over high heat, 6 to 7 minutes per side (less if you like your beef rare). Remove from grill, and let steak sit for 5 minutes. Slice thinly, making diagonal slices against the grain of the meat. Serve hot.

Makes 4 to 6 servings (about 4 to 6 ounces each).

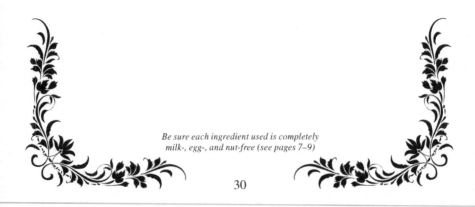

Be sure each ingredient used is completely milk-, egg-, and nut-free (see pages 7–9)

Flank Steak Yakitori

All the flavor of Beef Yakitori without all the work.

Preparation time: 5 minutes
Marinating time: 24 hours
Cooking time: 14 minutes

½ cup dairy-free **low-sodium soy sauce**
2 tablespoons pure cane sugar
2 tablespoons freshly squeezed lemon juice
½ teaspoon ground ginger
½ teaspoon bottled **minced garlic**
1 flank steak, about 1½ pounds

Place all ingredients except steak in a large sealable plastic bag. Seal
bag and shake to mix. Trim all fat from steak and then add steak to bag;
seal and shake to coat. Seal bag and refrigerate for 24 hours, turning
the bag over once about halfway through the marinating time.

To cook, either broil or grill.

To broil: Preheat broiler. Line broiler pan with aluminum foil. Place
marinated steak in prepared pan. Discard marinade. Broil for about
6 to 7 minutes per side (less if you like your beef rare). Remove from
broiler, and let steak sit for 5 minutes.

To grill: Preheat gas grill to high. Discard marinade. Grill steak over
high heat, 6 to 7 minutes per side (less if you like your beef rare).
Remove from grill, and let steak sit for 5 minutes.

Slice thinly, making diagonal slices against the grain of the meat.
Serve hot.

Makes 4 to 6 servings (about 4 to 6 ounces each).

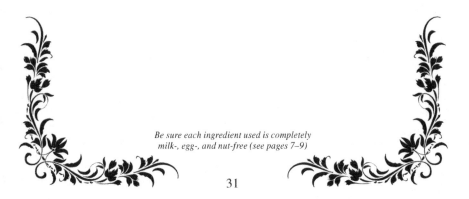

*Be sure each ingredient used is completely
milk-, egg-, and nut-free (see pages 7–9)*

Hot Dog Tidbits

*Although this is meant as an appetizer, I sometimes
like to make it as a dinner entrée, too.*

**Preparation time: 5 to 6 minutes
Cooking time: 20 minutes**

1 package of 7 dairy-, egg-, and nut-free **hot dogs** (preferably kosher
    hot dogs)
2 tablespoons water
1 tablespoon corn starch
½ cup seedless **blackberry jam** or **blackberry sugar-free fruit spread**
1 tablespoon **Worcestershire sauce**
1 tablespoon **ketchup**

Cut hot dogs into quarters.

Place corn starch and water in a small bowl; mix well and then set
aside. Place blackberry jam, Worcestershire sauce, and ketchup in a
2-quart saucepan. Bring to a boil over high heat, stirring frequently.
Add corn starch mixture; reduce heat to medium and cook, stirring
constantly, until mixture is thick enough to coat the hot dogs. Add
prepared hot dogs. Reduce heat to low and simmer, covered, for
20 minutes, stirring occasionally. Serve hot.

**Makes 7 appetizer servings (4 tidbits each) or
3 entrée servings (9 tidbits each).**

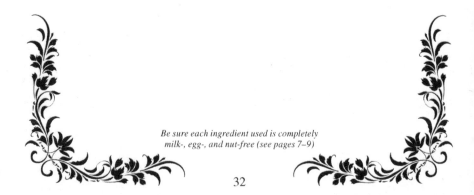

*Be sure each ingredient used is completely
milk-, egg-, and nut-free (see pages 7–9)*

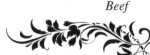

Jason's Four-Star Brisket

This is one of my son Jason's favorite foods, so I always try to keep some in the freezer for him to bring to social events. If you've never made brisket, keep in mind that this cut of meat shrinks up quite a bit while it cooks – which is why I say you will only get about 6 servings from a 3 pound piece of meat.

Preparation time: 15 minutes
Cooking time: 3½ hours

1 (12 ounce) bottle **chili sauce** (the type that is similar to ketchup, not the spicy variety with chile peppers)
¼ cup firmly packed pure cane dark brown sugar
1 tablespoon lemon juice (either freshly squeezed or bottled)
1 teaspoon bottled **minced garlic**
2 teaspoons dried rosemary, crumbled
2 teaspoons dried basil leaves
1 teaspoon paprika
3 pounds boneless flat-cut beef brisket roast (not corned beef brisket)*
salt and freshly ground black pepper, to taste
1 to 2 cups sherry wine

Preheat oven to 350 degrees F.

To make sauce place chili sauce, brown sugar, lemon juice, garlic, rosemary, basil leaves, and paprika in a 1- or 2-quart saucepan; mix well. Bring to a boil over high heat, stirring frequently. Cover and simmer over low heat for 5 minutes, stirring occasionally.

While sauce is simmering, trim all fat off of brisket and place in a 9-inch by 13-inch baking dish. Season on all sides with salt and pepper, and then baste on all sides with sauce. Pour sherry around, but not over, brisket, to a depth of ½ inch. Cover *tightly* with foil. Bake for 3 hours. Remove from oven and place brisket on a carving board. Slice against the grain into ¼-inch thick slices.

Place sliced brisket back into the baking dish. Spoon the sauce that is in the baking dish over the sliced meat, taking care to get the sauce both over and in between the slices. Cover baking dish tightly with foil and return to oven to cook for an additional 30 minutes. Place brisket on a serving platter and pour sauce into a gravy boat. Serve brisket hot, with sauce.

Makes 6 servings (about 3 or 4 slices each).

*Note: If you purchase a larger piece of meat you must increase the sauce quantity accordingly.

*Be sure each ingredient used is completely
milk-, egg-, and nut-free (see pages 7–9)*

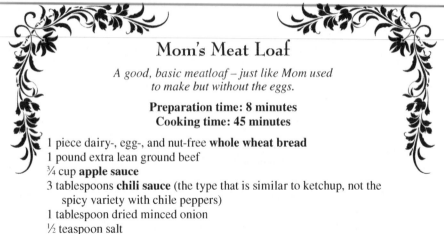

Mom's Meat Loaf

*A good, basic meatloaf – just like Mom used
to make but without the eggs.*

**Preparation time: 8 minutes
Cooking time: 45 minutes**

1 piece dairy-, egg-, and nut-free **whole wheat bread**
1 pound extra lean ground beef
¾ cup **apple sauce**
3 tablespoons **chili sauce** (the type that is similar to ketchup, not the
   spicy variety with chile peppers)
1 tablespoon dried minced onion
½ teaspoon salt
½ teaspoon **lemon pepper**

Heat oven to 400 degrees F.

Place bread in a blender or in a food processor that has been fitted
with the metal blade; process until bread turns into fine crumbs. Place
bread crumbs and remaining ingredients in a medium mixing bowl;
mix well.

Press meat mixture evenly into a 9-inch by 5-inch loaf pan. Bake for
about 45 minutes, or until done. Drain and discard fat. Serve hot.

Makes 4 servings (4 ounces each).

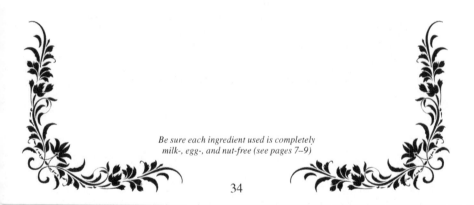

*Be sure each ingredient used is completely
milk-, egg-, and nut-free (see pages 7–9)*

Savory Herbed Steak

This steak is equally delicious cooked on the grill or in the broiler.

Preparation time: 5 minutes
Cooking time: 10 minutes

2 teaspoons dried basil leaves
2 teaspoons dried minced onion
1 teaspoon dried sage leaves
1 teaspoon dried oregano leaves
1 teaspoon paprika
½ teaspoon garlic salt
1½ pounds boneless steak, such as beef round, top round, or tri-tip steaks, cut 1-inch thick

Preheat gas grill or broiler.

Place all ingredients except steak in a small bowl; mix well. Sprinkle seasoning mixture evenly over both sides of steak, and then use your fingers to press the seasoning into the surface of the meat.

Grill over medium heat or broil for about 5 to 6 minutes per side, until cooked to desired doneness. Serve hot.

Makes 4 to 6 servings (4 to 6 ounces each).

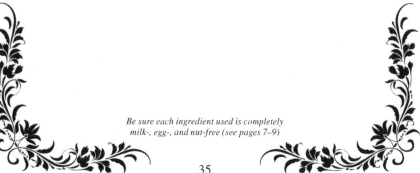

*Be sure each ingredient used is completely
milk-, egg-, and nut-free (see pages 7–9)*

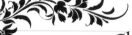

Sloppy Joe Wraps

These kid-pleasing wraps are perfect for a quick dinner or hot lunch.

Preparation and cooking time: 17 to 20 minutes

½ of a small zucchini
2 green onions (scallions)
1 pound extra lean ground beef
½ cup **chili sauce** (the type that is similar to ketchup, not the spicy
    variety with chile peppers)
3 tablespoons firmly packed pure cane dark brown sugar
6 (8-inch-diameter) **whole wheat tortillas**

Trim ends off zucchini. Finely chop zucchini; you should have ½ cup.
Thinly slice green onions (including green tops). Place ground beef
and prepared vegetables in a 12-inch skillet. Cook over medium-high
heat about 5 minutes or until beef is completely cooked through (with
no pink or red showing), stirring frequently and breaking beef into
small pieces as it cooks. Drain and discard fat.

In a small bowl or measuring cup, stir together chili sauce and brown
sugar; add to ground beef mixture and cook over medium-high heat
for 1 minute, stirring constantly. Remove skillet from heat.

Place tortillas on microwave-safe plate; microwave on high for
30 seconds or until warm. To assemble wraps spoon ½ cup of meat
mixture onto each tortilla. Fold bottom half of tortillas up, and then
fold each side in towards the center. Serve immediately.

Makes 3 to 6 servings (1 to 2 wraps each).

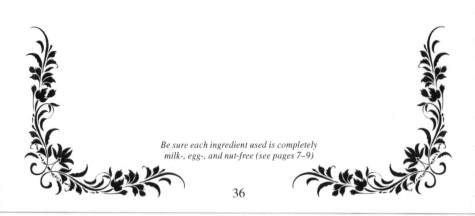

*Be sure each ingredient used is completely
milk-, egg-, and nut-free (see pages 7–9)*

Slow Cooker Beef with Rosemary and Potatoes

I'm beginning to wonder how I ever lived without a slow cooker. Now I like to plan ahead on those days when I know we'll be coming home late, tired and hungry. With about 15 minutes of effort (all of which can be done the night before), a "one pot" dinner is ready and waiting for us at the end of a long day.

Preparation time: 15 minutes
Cooking time: 8 hours

2¼ pounds boneless beef short ribs OR boneless beef chuck cross
    rib roast OR boneless beef top round roast
1 pound small white potatoes
3 large cloves fresh garlic
1 cup peeled baby-cut carrots
1 cup dairy-free **low-sodium beef broth**
½ cup Burgundy wine
3 tablespoons corn starch
1 tablespoon fresh rosemary leaves
¾ teaspoon salt
½ teaspoon pepper

Trim fat from beef and then cut beef into 1-inch cubes. Scrub potatoes and cut into pieces that are smaller than the beef cubes. Peel garlic and press through garlic press.

Place beef, potatoes, garlic, carrots, and beef broth in a 5-quart slow cooker. Place corn starch and wine in a small bowl or measuring cup; mix well and then pour over beef. Sprinkle with rosemary, salt, and pepper. Cover and cook on low heat setting for 8 hours.

Makes 4 servings (about 1⅔ cups each).

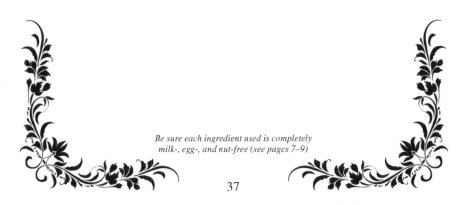

Be sure each ingredient used is completely milk-, egg-, and nut-free (see pages 7–9)

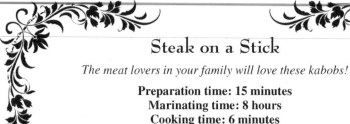

Steak on a Stick

The meat lovers in your family will love these kabobs!

Preparation time: 15 minutes
Marinating time: 8 hours
Cooking time: 6 minutes

1¾ pounds boneless top sirloin steak
3 tablespoons **orange juice**
2 tablespoons freshly squeezed lemon juice
1 tablespoon olive oil
1 tablespoon honey
1 tablespoon **Italian seasoning**
salt and freshly ground black pepper, to taste

Trim fat from steak and then cut steak into 1-inch cubes. Place remaining ingredients in a medium bowl; mix well. Add steak cubes to marinade in bowl; cover and refrigerate for at least 8 hours.

Preheat gas grill. While grill is heating, skewer meat onto five 10-inch-long metal skewers, leaving ¼-inch of space between the pieces of meat.

Grill for 3 minutes over high heat; turn over and grill for an additional 2 or 3 minutes, until cooked to desired doneness. Serve hot.

Makes 5 servings (1 skewer each).

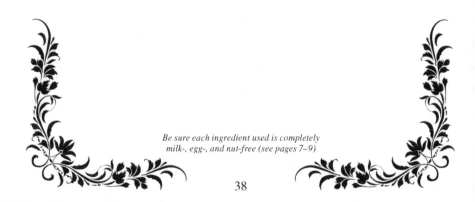

*Be sure each ingredient used is completely
milk-, egg-, and nut-free (see pages 7–9)*

Stir-Fried Beef with Broccoli

*As with any stir-fry recipe, be sure to avoid using a
wok that has been "seasoned" with peanut oil.*

Preparation and cooking time: 30 minutes

¼ cup dairy-free **low-sodium soy sauce**
¼ cup sherry wine
2 teaspoons pure cane sugar
1 teaspoon bottled **minced ginger**
1 teaspoon bottled **minced garlic**
2 teaspoons corn starch
¾ cup + 2 tablespoons water, divided use
⅔ pound fresh broccoli crowns
1 pound boneless top sirloin steak
1 tablespoon canola or **vegetable oil**

To make sauce, place soy sauce, sherry, sugar, ginger, and garlic in
a medium bowl; mix well and then set aside. Place corn starch and
2 tablespoons water in a small bowl; mix well and then set aside.

Cut broccoli into small florets; set aside. Trim all fat off steak; thinly
slice steak and then cut these slices into 1½-inch-long pieces. Add meat
to sauce in bowl; mix well.

Heat oil in wok over high heat. Add broccoli and stir-fry 2 minutes.
Add remaining ¾ cup water and bring to a boil. Reduce heat to medium
and simmer, covered, for about 3 to 5 minutes, until broccoli is slightly
tender. Remove broccoli from wok and place on a serving platter.
Discard water from wok.

Increase heat back to high. Using a slotted spoon, transfer meat to wok,
reserving sauce. Stir-fry 2 to 3 minutes, until meat is browned and
cooked through. Do not overcook. Remove meat from wok and place
on the serving platter. Place reserved sauce in wok. Bring to a boil
over high heat and then boil for 2 minutes. Add corn starch mixture
and cook over high heat, stirring constantly, until sauce thickens. Pour
sauce over meat and broccoli on serving platter; mix well. Serve hot.

Makes 4 servings (about ¾ cup each).

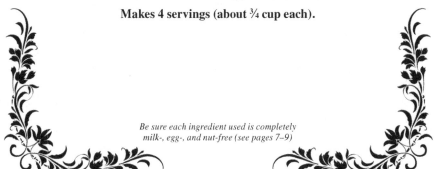

*Be sure each ingredient used is completely
milk-, egg-, and nut-free (see pages 7–9)*

Stir-Fried Beef with Sugar Snap Peas

This has become a real favorite in the Coss household.

Preparation time: 13 minutes
Marinating time: 30 minutes
Cooking time: 5 minutes

⅓ cup pineapple juice
¼ cup dairy-free **low-sodium soy sauce**
1 teaspoon dairy-, egg-, and nut-free **Worcestershire sauce**
½ teaspoon bottled **minced garlic**
1 pound boneless London broil steak
½ pound fresh sugar snap peas
1 tablespoon canola or **vegetable oil**
1 tablespoon corn starch

To make marinade place pineapple juice, soy sauce, Worcestershire sauce, and garlic in a medium bowl; mix well and then set aside.

Trim all fat off steak; slice steak into ¼-inch-thick strips and then slice each strip into 1-inch-long pieces. Add beef to marinade in bowl; toss to coat. Cover and refrigerate for at least 30 minutes, up to 24 hours.

Wash and trim peas; set aside.

After the beef has marinated, heat oil in wok over high heat. Add peas and 1 tablespoon of the sauce to wok. Stir-fry about 1½ minutes. Remove peas from wok and place on a serving platter.

Using a slotted spoon, add marinated beef (without sauce) to wok. Stir-fry about 3 minutes, until cooked through. Using a slotted spoon, remove cooked beef from wok and place on the serving platter. Stir corn starch into remaining marinade, and then add to pan juices in wok. Cook, stirring constantly, until the sauce comes to a boil and thickens. Pour sauce over cooked beef and peas on serving platter; toss gently to coat. Serve hot.

Makes 4 servings (about 1 cup each).

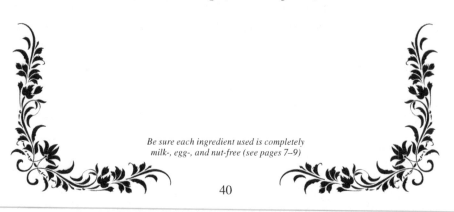

*Be sure each ingredient used is completely
milk-, egg-, and nut-free (see pages 7–9)*

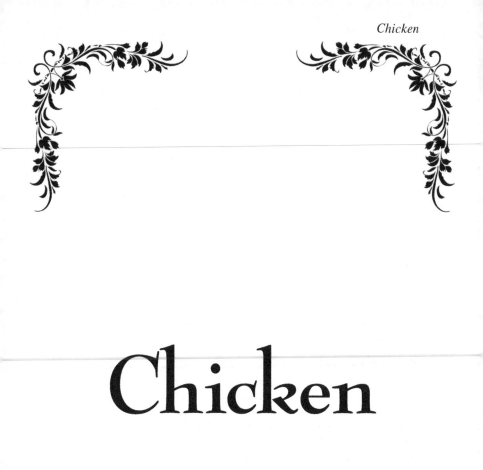

Chicken

Best-Loved Roasted Chicken Dinner

*This makes the house smell so good your family will be
clamoring for dinner. You may even want to make 2 chickens
and save the leftovers for sandwiches and salads.*

Preparation time: 10 minutes
Cooking time: 1½ hours

1 roasting chicken, about 4½ pounds
1 small brown onion
salt and pepper
2 sprigs fresh rosemary
2 sprigs fresh parsley
2 sprigs fresh thyme
¼ cup olive oil
¼ cup **orange juice**
½ teaspoon onion salt
1½ pound potatoes (any variety)
1 (1-pound) bag peeled baby-cut carrots

Preheat oven to 400 degrees F.

Remove giblets from chicken; either discard or save for another use.
Wash chicken inside and out; pat dry with paper towels. Peel onion and
cut into quarters. Sprinkle inside of chicken with salt and pepper. Place
quartered onion and herb sprigs into chicken cavity. Place chicken in a
large roasting pan, breast side up.

Place oil, orange juice, and onion salt in a small bowl or measuring cup;
mix well. Brush chicken on all sides with some of the olive oil mixture.
Bake for 30 minutes.

Meanwhile, scrub potatoes and cut into 1-inch pieces.

Remove chicken from oven. Add potatoes and carrots to the roasting
pan. Baste chicken and vegetables with olive oil mixture. Bake for
another 30 minutes. Baste with olive oil mixture or pan drippings, and
then bake for an additional 30 minutes or until the internal temperature
of the chicken registers 175 degrees on a meat thermometer and the
vegetables feel tender when pierced with a fork. Serve hot.

Makes 4 servings.

*Be sure each ingredient used is completely
milk-, egg-, and nut-free (see pages 7–9)*

Chicken Marsala

*By starting with thin-sliced chicken breast filets
and pre-sliced mushrooms you can have an elegant
entrée on the table in only 20 minutes.*

Preparation and cooking time: 20 minutes

¼ cup **all-purpose flour**
2 teaspoons **Italian seasoning**, divided use
1 pound thin-sliced chicken breast filets
2 tablespoons olive oil
1 tablespoon dairy-free **margarine**
1 (6 ounce) package sliced fresh button mushrooms
salt and freshly ground pepper, to taste
1 (14½ ounce) can **diced and peeled tomatoes in tomato juice**,
    drained
½ cup **Marsala cooking wine**
1 tablespoon corn starch
2 tablespoons water

Place flour and 1 teaspoon Italian seasoning in a shallow dish; mix well
and then set aside. Rinse chicken in water, and then dip the wet chicken
pieces into the flour mixture to coat on both sides.

Heat oil in a 12-inch non-stick skillet over high heat. Place the coated
chicken in a single layer in the skillet. Cover and cook until lightly
browned, about 3 minutes. Turn the chicken over and cook, covered,
for another 3 to 4 minutes, until chicken is cooked through. Remove the
chicken from the skillet and place on a serving platter.

To make sauce, melt margarine in the same 12-inch skillet over
medium-high heat. Add sliced mushrooms, remaining 1 teaspoon
Italian seasoning, salt, and pepper and sauté for about 3 minutes,
stirring frequently, until mushrooms are somewhat soft. Stir in
tomatoes and Marsala wine; bring to a boil over high heat. Place corn
starch and water in a small bowl; mix well and then add to boiling
sauce. Cook, stirring constantly, until sauce thickens. Spoon sauce over
cooked chicken. Serve immediately.

Makes 4 servings.

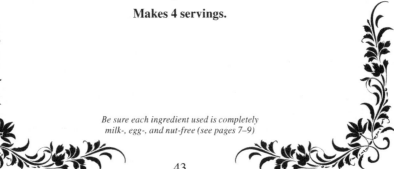

*Be sure each ingredient used is completely
milk-, egg-, and nut-free (see pages 7–9)*

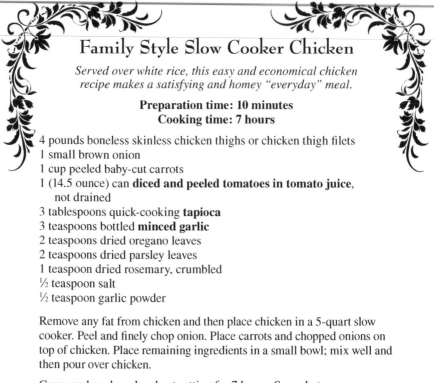

Family Style Slow Cooker Chicken

Served over white rice, this easy and economical chicken recipe makes a satisfying and homey "everyday" meal.

Preparation time: 10 minutes
Cooking time: 7 hours

4 pounds boneless skinless chicken thighs or chicken thigh filets
1 small brown onion
1 cup peeled baby-cut carrots
1 (14.5 ounce) can **diced and peeled tomatoes in tomato juice**, not drained
3 tablespoons quick-cooking **tapioca**
3 teaspoons bottled **minced garlic**
2 teaspoons dried oregano leaves
2 teaspoons dried parsley leaves
1 teaspoon dried rosemary, crumbled
½ teaspoon salt
½ teaspoon garlic powder

Remove any fat from chicken and then place chicken in a 5-quart slow cooker. Peel and finely chop onion. Place carrots and chopped onions on top of chicken. Place remaining ingredients in a small bowl; mix well and then pour over chicken.

Cover and cook on low heat setting for 7 hours. Serve hot.

Makes 6 servings.

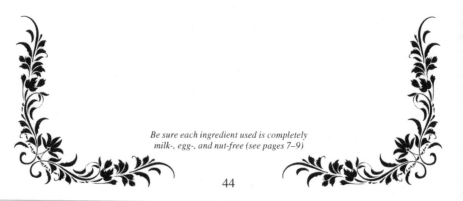

Be sure each ingredient used is completely milk-, egg-, and nut-free (see pages 7–9)

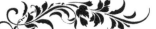

Four Ingredient Chicken

*Too tired to cook? Don't worry! Pair up this easy chicken with a
fresh green salad for a simple, elegant, and fuss-free dinner.*

Preparation time: 7 minutes
Cooking time: 35 minutes

4 boneless skinless chicken breast halves
¼ cup olive oil
2 tablespoons dairy- and egg-free **Dijon mustard**
1 tablespoon chopped fresh rosemary leaves

Preheat oven to 400 degrees F. Lightly spray a 9-inch by 13-inch baking
pan with dairy-free **non-stick cooking spray.**

Place oil and mustard in a small bowl or measuring cup; mix well with
a fork or small wire whisk. Place chicken in a single layer in prepared
pan. Brush mustard mixture onto both sides of chicken. Chop rosemary
and sprinkle over chicken. Bake, uncovered, for 35 minutes or until
juices run clear when chicken is pierced with a fork. Serve hot.

Makes 4 servings (1 chicken breast half each).

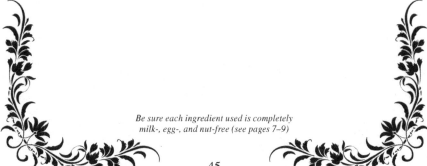

*Be sure each ingredient used is completely
milk-, egg-, and nut-free (see pages 7–9)*

Fried Chicken Tenders

A very kid-pleasing entrée that's easier to make than you might think. If your children would rather have chicken "nuggets," just cut each chicken tender into bite-size pieces before cooking, and then coat and cook as directed.

Preparation and cooking time: 30 minutes

¼ cup **vanilla-flavored soy milk** or **rice milk**
½ cup **all-purpose flour**
1 teaspoon dried basil leaves
1 teaspoon dried parsley leaves
¾ teaspoon salt
½ teaspoon pepper
1½ pounds chicken filet tenders
½ cup canola or **vegetable oil**

Place soy or rice milk in a shallow bowl. Place flour, basil, parsley, salt, and pepper in a second shallow bowl; mix well.

Line a serving platter with paper towels; set aside.

Rinse chicken but do not pat dry. Dip each chicken piece in the soy or rice milk and then in the flour mixture, coating both sides with the flour mixture; set aside.

Heat oil in a 12-inch skillet over medium-high heat. Place half of the prepared chicken tenders in a single layer in the skillet. Cook, covered with a wire "splatter guard," for 3 to 4 minutes or until the bottom of each piece of chicken turns golden brown. Turn chicken tenders over and cook an additional 3 minutes, or until cooked through. Place on prepared platter. Repeat with remaining chicken pieces. Serve immediately.

Makes 4 servings (about 4 chicken tenders each).

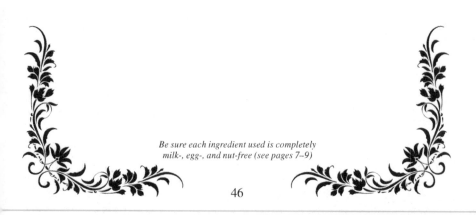

Be sure each ingredient used is completely milk-, egg-, and nut-free (see pages 7–9)

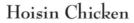

Hoisin Chicken

*Add some fresh steamed vegetables and sliced melon,
and you'll have a healthy and delicious dinner
on the table in about 30 minutes.*

**Preparation time: 7 minutes
Cooking time: 22 minutes**

6 boneless skinless chicken breast halves
½ cup dairy-, egg-, and nut-free **hoisin sauce** (available in the "Asian"
    section of the supermarket)
2 tablespoons firmly packed pure cane dark brown sugar
1 tablespoon **ketchup**
1 teaspoon bottled **minced garlic**
½ teaspoon bottled **minced ginger**

Preheat broiler. Spray rack of broiler pan with dairy-free **non-stick cooking spray**.

Place chicken in a single layer on the prepared pan. To make sauce place remaining ingredients in a small bowl; mix well. Brush sauce on one side of the chicken. Broil 10 minutes. Turn chicken over and brush with remaining sauce. Broil an additional 10 to 12 minutes, or until juices run clear when chicken is pierced with a fork. Serve hot.

Make 6 servings (1 chicken breast half each).

*Be sure each ingredient used is completely
milk-, egg-, and nut-free (see pages 7–9)*

Jammin' Chicken

The apricot jam and whole wheat bread give this chicken entrée a wonderful sweetness that kids love. But just make enough for today's meal, as the coating will be soggy and unappealing by tomorrow.

Preparation time: 8 minutes
Cooking time: 35 minutes

⅓ cup **apricot jam** or **apricot preserves**
2 slices dairy-, egg-, and nut-free **whole wheat bread**
4 boneless skinless chicken breast halves

Preheat oven to 375 degrees F. Spray a 9-inch by 13-inch baking pan with dairy-free **non-stick cooking spray.**

Place jam on a microwave-safe plate. Microwave on high for 30 to 45 seconds or until melted; stir. Place bread in a blender or a food processor that has been fitted with the metal blade and process on high until bread crumbs are as fine as they will get; place on a second plate.

Wash chicken and pat dry with paper towels. Coat both sides of each chicken piece with melted jam and then with bread crumbs; place in a single layer in the prepared baking pan. Bake for 35 minutes or until juices run clear when chicken is pierced with a fork. Serve immediately.

Makes 4 servings (1 chicken breast half each).

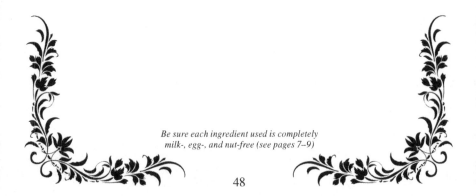

Be sure each ingredient used is completely milk-, egg-, and nut-free (see pages 7–9)

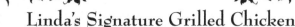

Linda's Signature Grilled Chicken

You're going to love this recipe! This amazingly easy chicken dish has become one of my summertime standards, enjoyed by my friends, my children, and my friends' children.

Preparation time: 3 minutes
Marinating time: 30 minutes
Cooking time: 16 to 20 minutes

¼ cup **balsamic vinegar**
2 tablespoons olive oil
½ tablespoon freshly squeezed lemon juice
½ teaspoon **lemon pepper**
4 boneless skinless chicken breast halves
canola or **vegetable oil** for brushing on grill

Place vinegar, oil, lemon juice, and lemon pepper in a small bowl or measuring cup; mix well. Place chicken in a single layer in a large sealable plastic bag; add marinade. Seal bag and shake gently to coat. Refrigerate 15 minutes. Turn bag over, keeping chicken in a single layer. Refrigerate for an additional 15 minutes. (Note: If desired, can be marinated up to 24 hours).

Heat gas grill, then brush grill with oil.

Place marinated chicken on prepared grill of heated barbecue. Discard excess marinade. Cover barbecue and cook for 8 to 10 minutes (note: If using a gas barbecue, cook over medium heat). Turn chicken over. Cover and cook for an additional 8 to 10 minutes, until juices run clear when chicken is pierced with a fork. Serve hot.

Makes 4 servings (1 chicken breast half each).

Note: Although this chicken is fabulous from the grill, it is not particularly good broiled. So if you live in a cold climate, save this recipe for barbecue season.

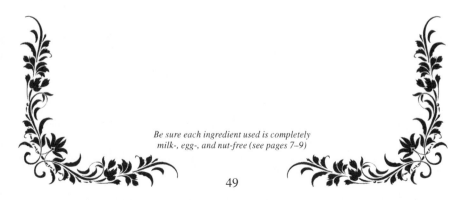

*Be sure each ingredient used is completely
milk-, egg-, and nut-free (see pages 7–9)*

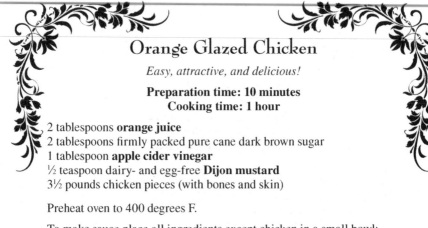

Orange Glazed Chicken

Easy, attractive, and delicious!

Preparation time: 10 minutes
Cooking time: 1 hour

2 tablespoons **orange juice**
2 tablespoons firmly packed pure cane dark brown sugar
1 tablespoon **apple cider vinegar**
½ teaspoon dairy- and egg-free **Dijon mustard**
3½ pounds chicken pieces (with bones and skin)

Preheat oven to 400 degrees F.

To make sauce place all ingredients except chicken in a small bowl; mix well.

Line a 9-inch by 13-inch baking dish with aluminum foil. Place chicken, skin side up, in a single layer on baking dish; brush with orange juice mixture. Bake for 1 hour or until juices run clear when chicken is pierced with a fork, basting with the orange juice mixture twice during the cooking time. Serve hot.

Makes 6 servings.

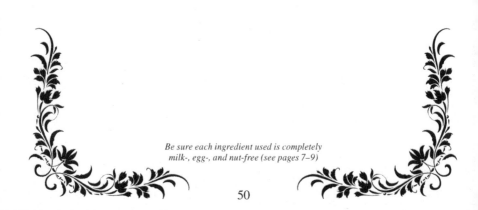

*Be sure each ingredient used is completely
milk-, egg-, and nut-free (see pages 7–9)*

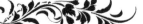

Plum Sauced Chicken in Tortillas

These wraps are practically a meal in themselves,
perfect for lunch or a light dinner.

Preparation time: 15 minutes
Cooking time: 30 minutes

1 (7 or 8 ounce) bottle dairy-, egg-, and nut-free **hoisin sauce**
   (available in the "Asian" section of the supermarket)
2 (3.5 ounce) containers **pureed peaches** (i.e., baby food)
½ cup **applesauce**
3 tablespoons quick-cooking **tapioca**
1 tablespoon **Chinese 5-Spice Powder**
½ tablespoon bottled **minced ginger**
3 pounds boneless, skinless chicken thighs and/or breasts
4 cups packaged **broccoli slaw**
12 (8-inch-diameter) **flour tortillas**, either room temperature or
   warmed

Place hoisin sauce, pureed peaches, applesauce, tapioca, Chinese
5-Spice Powder, and ginger in a 4-quart pot; mix well. Cut chicken into
2-inch-long strips; add to pot. Bring to a boil over high heat, stirring
occasionally. Reduce heat to low and simmer, covered, for 30 minutes,
stirring occasionally.

Place about ½ cup cooked chicken mixture and ⅓ cup broccoli slaw in
center of each tortilla. Fold up bottom edge of tortilla, and then fold in
each side. Serve immediately.

Makes 6 servings (2 wraps each).

Variation:

Slow Cooker
Plum Sauced Chicken in Tortillas

Preparation time: 15 minutes
Cooking time: 5 hours

Cut chicken into 2-inch-long strips; place in a 5-quart slow cooker.
Place hoisin sauce, pureed peaches, applesauce, tapioca, Chinese
5-Spice Powder, and ginger in a medium bowl; mix well and then
pour over chicken. Cover and cook on low heat setting for 5 hours.
Assemble tortillas as directed above.

Be sure each ingredient used is completely
milk-, egg-, and nut-free (see pages 7–9)

51

Seasoned Baked Chicken

Seasoned and baked chicken has been a favorite of mine for many years. Here I present you with basic cooking instructions for Seasoned Baked Chicken and a number of different suggestions for seasoning combinations. You just need to decide how much chicken you want to cook, pick a seasoning blend, cook, and enjoy!

Preparation time: depends on quantity of chicken to wash
Cooking time: 1 hour

cut-up chicken pieces (with bones and skin)
canola or olive oil
seasonings

Preheat oven to 350 or 375 degrees F. Line a shallow baking dish with aluminum foil. Place washed chicken, skin side down, in a single layer on the prepared baking dish. Using a pastry brush, brush chicken with oil. Sprinkle generously with each seasoning that is in the desired seasoning combination. Turn chicken over, brush with oil, and sprinkle with seasonings. Bake, uncovered, for about 1 hour or until juices run clear when chicken is pierced with a fork.

Seasoning Combination #1
I prefer this with mild curry powder, but your family may like things spicier.

curry powder
garlic powder
lemon pepper

Seasoning Combination #2
Simple and flavorful.

ground sage
ground ginger
ground mustard powder
turmeric
salt and pepper, to taste

Seasoning Combination #3
Try sprinkling the garlic salt on first and fairly heavily, and then top things off with just a light sprinkling of the nutmeg.

garlic salt
ground sage
ground oregano
ground marjoram
celery seed
black pepper
ground nutmeg

Seasoning Combination #4
This combination tastes best when the chicken is brushed with olive oil rather than canola.

ground mustard powder
ground sage
ground marjoram
dried rosemary, crumbled
salt

*Be sure each ingredient used is completely
milk-, egg-, and nut-free (see pages 7–9)*

Stir-Fried Chicken with Asparagus

Chicken, asparagus, and a flavorful sauce combine for a great stir-fry.

Preparation time: 10 minutes
Cooking time: 15 minutes

⅓ cup dairy-free **low-sodium soy sauce**
⅓ cup **orange juice**
¼ cup **red wine vinegar**
1 tablespoon freshly squeezed lemon juice
1 tablespoon pure cane sugar
1 teaspoon sesame oil
1 teaspoon bottled **minced ginger**
1 teaspoon bottled **minced garlic**
4 boneless, skinless chicken breast halves
1 pound fresh asparagus
¾ cup chopped onion
1 tablespoon canola or **vegetable oil**
2 tablespoons corn starch

Place soy sauce, orange juice, vinegar, lemon juice, sugar, sesame oil, ginger, and garlic in a medium bowl; mix well. Cut chicken into ¾-inch chunks; add to the bowl with the sauce.

Remove and discard woody ends from asparagus, and then cut asparagus into 1-inch-long pieces. Peel and chop onion.

Heat oil in wok over high heat. Add prepared asparagus; stir-fry 2 to 3 minutes (depending on thickness of asparagus stalks). Add chopped onion; stir-fry an additional 2 minutes. Remove asparagus and onion from wok and place on a serving platter.

Using a slotted spoon, add half of marinated chicken pieces to wok; stir-fry about 3 to 4 minutes, until cooked through. Remove from wok and place on the serving platter. Repeat with remaining chicken.

Place remaining sauce in wok and bring to a boil. Reduce heat to low. Using a fork or wire whisk, stir in corn starch. Cook over low heat, stirring constantly, until sauce thickens. Pour sauce over chicken and vegetables on serving platter; stir to coat. Serve hot, over steamed rice.

Makes 4 servings (about 1¼ cups each).

*Be sure each ingredient used is completely
milk-, egg-, and nut-free (see pages 7–9)*

Wonderful Winter Chicken

*Get out your slow cooker to make this family-pleasing
chicken that's perfect for a cold winter night.*

**Preparation time: 15 minutes
Cooking time: 8 hours**

4 pounds boneless skinless chicken thighs
1 medium brown onion
1 (6 or 8 ounce) package fresh sliced button mushrooms
⅔ cup Burgundy wine
¼ cup firmly packed pure cane dark brown sugar
1 tablespoon finely grated lemon peel
3 teaspoons bottled **minced garlic**
2 teaspoons dried basil leaves
1 teaspoon dried oregano leaves
1 teaspoon **seasoned salt**
freshly ground black pepper, to taste

Trim fat from chicken and then place chicken pieces into a 5-quart
slow cooker. Peel and chop onion. Place chopped onion and sliced
mushrooms on top of chicken. Combine remaining ingredients in a
small mixing bowl and then add to slow cooker. Cover and cook on low
heat setting for 8 hours. Serve hot.

Makes 6 servings.

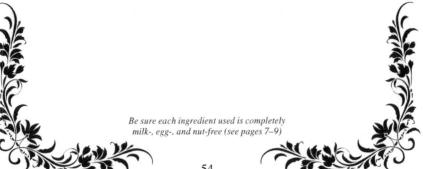

*Be sure each ingredient used is completely
milk-, egg-, and nut-free (see pages 7–9)*

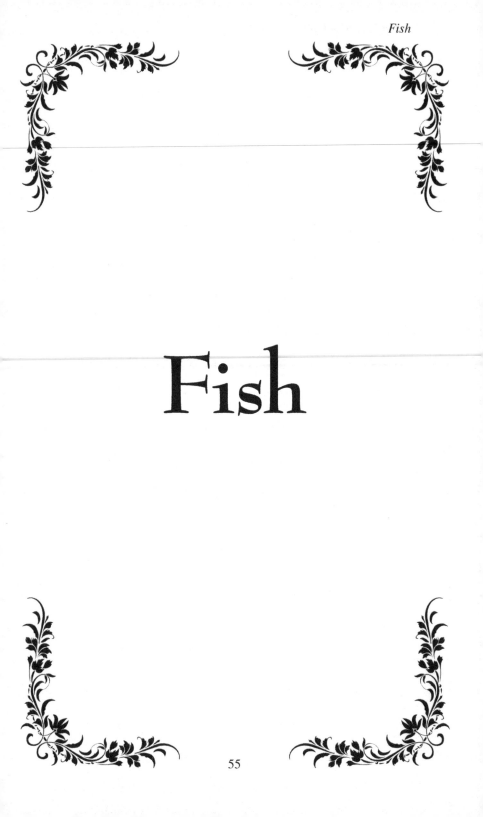

Fish

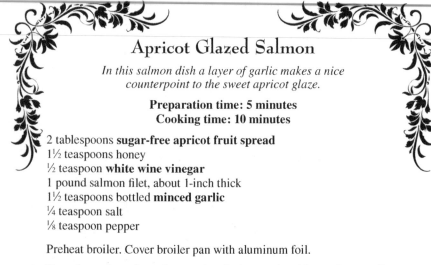

Apricot Glazed Salmon

*In this salmon dish a layer of garlic makes a nice
counterpoint to the sweet apricot glaze.*

Preparation time: 5 minutes
Cooking time: 10 minutes

2 tablespoons **sugar-free apricot fruit spread**
1½ teaspoons honey
½ teaspoon **white wine vinegar**
1 pound salmon filet, about 1-inch thick
1½ teaspoons bottled **minced garlic**
¼ teaspoon salt
⅛ teaspoon pepper

Preheat broiler. Cover broiler pan with aluminum foil.

To make apricot glaze place apricot fruit spread and honey in a small
microwave-safe bowl. Microwave on high for 30 seconds or until
liquefied; stir in vinegar and then set aside.

Place salmon, skin side down, on prepared broiler pan. Place garlic,
salt, and pepper in a small bowl; mix well and then spread evenly over
salmon. Broil for 6 minutes. Spread apricot glaze evenly over salmon.
Broil for an additional 4 minutes or until done; serve immediately.

Makes 4 servings (4 ounces each).

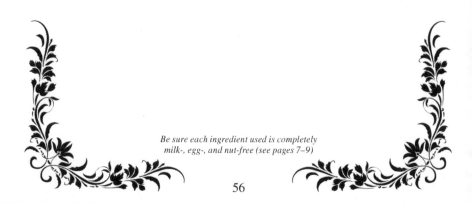

*Be sure each ingredient used is completely
milk-, egg-, and nut-free (see pages 7–9)*

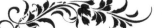

Easy Baked Salmon

Slow baking allows the flavors of the sweet sauce to permeate the fish.

Preparation time: 5 minutes
Cooking time: 35 to 40 minutes

1 green onion (scallion)
1 pound boneless skinless salmon filet, about 1-inch thick
3 tablespoons honey
1 tablespoon dairy-free **low-sodium soy sauce**
1 teaspoon bottled **minced garlic**

Preheat oven to 350 degrees F. Spray a baking pan with dairy-free **non-stick cooking spray.**

Mince green onion; set aside.

Place salmon in prepared pan. Place honey, soy sauce, and garlic in a small bowl; mix well. Brush salmon with half of sauce. Bake for 20 minutes. Brush salmon with remaining sauce and sprinkle with the minced green onion. Bake for an additional 15 to 20 minutes or until done. Serve immediately.

Makes 4 servings (4 ounces each).

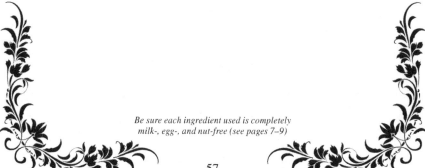

*Be sure each ingredient used is completely
milk-, egg-, and nut-free (see pages 7–9)*

Fast and Easy Red Snapper

*One of the things I love about fish is how
quick and easy it is to prepare.*

Preparation and cooking time: 15 minutes

⅓ cup **whole wheat flour**
1 teaspoon dried parsley leaves
1 teaspoon dried oregano leaves
freshly ground black pepper to taste
¼ cup dairy-free **margarine**, divided use
1 pound fresh red snapper filets
2 tablespoons freshly squeezed lemon juice
1 teaspoon bottled **minced ginger**

Place flour, parsley, oregano, and pepper in a shallow dish; mix well.
Rinse fish in water, and then dip the wet fish filets in the flour mixture
to coat both sides

Heat 2 tablespoons margarine in a 12-inch skillet over medium-high
heat. Place coated fish filets in a single layer in skillet. Cook for
2½ minutes per side, until done. Using a slotted wide spatula, remove
cooked fish from skillet and place on a serving platter.

Reduce heat to low. Add lemon juice, ginger, and the remaining
2 tablespoons margarine to the skillet. Cook, stirring constantly, until
margarine melts. Drizzle sauce over fish and serve immediately.

Makes 4 servings (4 ounces each).

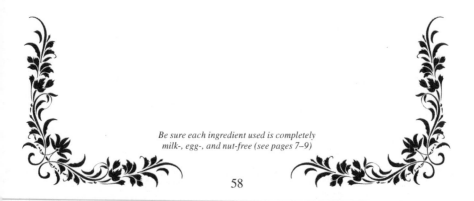

*Be sure each ingredient used is completely
milk-, egg-, and nut-free (see pages 7–9)*

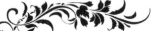

Mandarin Sole

*Filet of sole cooks very quickly, so keep a close eye
on these to make sure they don't overcook.*

Preparation and cooking time: 18 minutes

2 tablespoons water
1 tablespoon corn starch
2 tablespoons dairy-free **low-sodium soy sauce**
2 tablespoons sherry wine
1 tablespoon **red wine vinegar**
1 teaspoon sesame oil
2 teaspoons bottled **minced ginger**
½ teaspoon pure cane sugar
2 tablespoons dairy-free **margarine**
1¼ pounds filet of sole

To make sauce, mix water with corn starch and then set aside. Place soy
sauce, sherry, vinegar, sesame oil, ginger, and sugar in a 1- or 2-quart
saucepan; mix well. Bring to a boil over high heat. Reduce heat to low
and add corn starch mixture. Stir constantly until sauce thickens, about
1 minute; set aside.

Melt margarine in a 12-inch skillet over medium-high heat. Place half
of fish filets in a single layer in the skillet. Cook about 2 to 3 minutes
per side, until cooked through. Remove fish from skillet and place on a
serving platter. Repeat with remaining fish. Pour sauce over cooked fish
and serve immediately.

Makes 4 servings (5 ounces each).

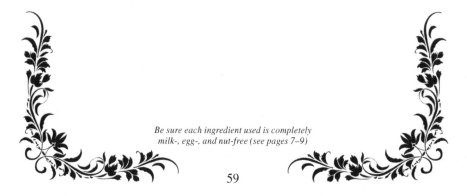

*Be sure each ingredient used is completely
milk-, egg-, and nut-free (see pages 7–9)*

Marinated Orange Roughy

*If orange roughy isn't available you can try this with
cod, haddock, or another variety of white fish.*

Preparation time: 3 minutes
Marinating time: 2 hours
Cooking time: 4 to 8 minutes

3 tablespoons lime juice
2 tablespoons olive oil
1 teaspoon dried thyme leaves
1 teaspoon bottled **minced ginger**
⅛ teaspoon salt
1 pound orange roughy filets

To make marinade place lime juice, olive oil, thyme, minced ginger,
and salt in a small bowl or measuring cup; mix well. Place orange
roughy in a large sealable plastic bag; add marinade. Seal bag and
shake gently to coat. Refrigerate 1 hour. Turn bag over and then
refrigerate for an additional hour.

Preheat broiler. Spray rack of broiler pan with dairy-free **non-stick
cooking spray.** Place orange roughy on the prepared pan. Brush with
some of the extra marinade from the bag. Broil for approximately 2 to
4 minutes per side, until done. Serve hot.

Makes 4 servings (4 ounces each).

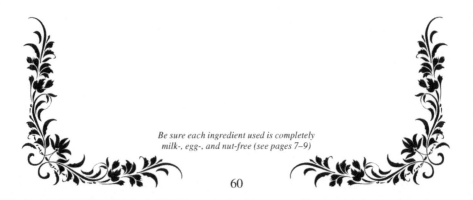

*Be sure each ingredient used is completely
milk-, egg-, and nut-free (see pages 7–9)*

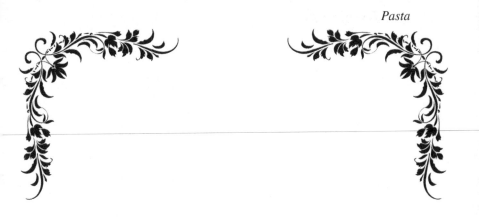

Pasta

Farmer's Market Pasta

This light and healthy pasta dish was inspired by the bounty of fresh vegetables available at my local farmer's market.

Preparation and cooking time: 25 to 30 minutes

1 (8 ounce) package dairy-, egg-, and nut-free **penne pasta** (skinny tube-shaped pasta)
1 small ear corn on the cob
2 small or 1 medium zucchini
1 small yellow squash
1 medium tomato
½ of a medium-size red bell pepper
1 cup firmly packed fresh basil leaves
4 medium cloves fresh garlic
3 tablespoons olive oil, divided use
salt and freshly ground black pepper, to taste

Prepare pasta according to the package directions; drain.

While pasta is cooking, prepare vegetables. Cut corn off the cob. Trim ends off zucchini and yellow squash and then cut zucchini and yellow squash into approximately 1½- to 2-inch-long by ¼-inch-thick matchsticks. Seed and chop tomato. Seed bell pepper, cut into thin strips, and then cut strips into approximately 1½-inch-long pieces. Chop basil. Peel garlic and press through garlic press.

Heat 1 tablespoon olive oil in a 12-inch skillet over medium-high heat. Add prepared vegetables, basil, and garlic. Sauté over medium-high heat, stirring frequently, for about 7 minutes or until vegetables are cooked.

Place cooked pasta, cooked vegetables, remaining 2 tablespoons olive oil, salt, and pepper in a large serving bowl; mix well. Serve hot.

Makes 6 servings (about 1 cup each).

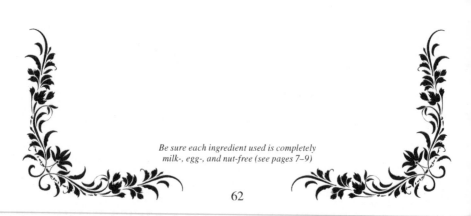

Be sure each ingredient used is completely milk-, egg-, and nut-free (see pages 7–9)

Fruited Pasta Salad

This makes a terrific side dish to serve with grilled chicken or steak, and is easily doubled to feed a crowd.

Preparation time: 4 minutes
Cooking time: 20 minutes
Refrigeration time: 4 hours or more

1 (8 ounce) package dairy-, egg-, and nut-free **large elbow macaroni**
3 tablespoons olive oil
3 tablespoons apple juice
1½ tablespoons **balsamic vinegar**
1 teaspoon ground cinnamon
½ teaspoon dairy- and egg-free **Dijon mustard**
⅛ teaspoon salt
⅛ teaspoon pepper
2 (11 ounce) cans **mandarin oranges**, drained
½ cup **golden raisins**

Prepare pasta according to the package directions; drain.

While pasta is cooking, make dressing. Place olive oil, apple juice, vinegar, cinnamon, mustard, salt, and pepper in a small bowl; mix well.

Place cooked and drained pasta in a large serving bowl. Add prepared dressing, mandarin oranges, and raisins; toss gently. Cover and refrigerate until cold, about 4 hours. Serve cold.

Makes 6 servings (1 cup each).

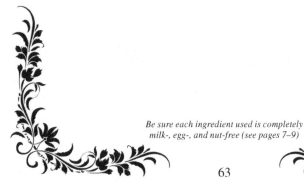

Be sure each ingredient used is completely milk-, egg-, and nut-free (see pages 7–9)

Lemony Pasta Primavera with Salmon

*Fresh salmon, vegetables, and lemon combine to make
a very attractive dish that's a meal in itself.*

Preparation and cooking time: 35 minutes

1 (12 ounce) package dairy-, egg-, and nut-free **penne pasta** (skinny tube-shaped pasta)
1 pound boneless, skinless fresh salmon filet
1 cup sherry wine
2 lemons
1 pound fresh asparagus, preferably fairly thin
1 cup peeled baby-cut carrots
4 green onions (scallions)
1 tablespoon olive oil
½ cup **julienne-sliced sun-dried tomatoes packed in oil**, drained
3 tablespoons dairy-free **margarine**, melted
½ teaspoon salt
½ teaspoon pepper

Prepare pasta according to the package directions; drain.

While pasta is cooking, slice salmon crosswise into ¼-inch-wide strips. Cut each strip into 2-inch-long pieces. Place salmon pieces in a single layer in a 12-inch skillet. Add sherry. Bring to a boil over high heat and then reduce heat to low and simmer, covered, for 5 minutes or until salmon is cooked through. Using a slotted spatula, remove salmon from skillet and place on a plate; set aside. Discard liquid from skillet.

While salmon is cooking, begin to prepare lemon and vegetables. Finely grate 2 tablespoons of lemon peel and squeeze ¼ cup of fresh lemon juice; place in a small bowl and set aside. Remove and discard woody ends from asparagus, and cut asparagus into 2-inch-long pieces. Cut carrots lengthwise into quarters. Slice green onions (both green and white parts) into 2-inch-long pieces.

Once salmon is cooked and skillet is empty, place oil in skillet and heat over high heat. Add carrots and asparagus and sauté for about 4 minutes, just until vegetables are slightly tender. Add green onion and sauté for an additional 3 minutes. Remove skillet from heat. Stir in sun-dried tomatoes.

Add melted margarine, salt, and pepper to the lemon peel and juice in the small bowl; mix well. Place drained pasta, cooked salmon, cooked vegetables, and margarine mixture in a large serving bowl; toss gently. Serve immediately.

Makes 6 servings (about 2 cups each).

*Be sure each ingredient used is completely
milk-, egg-, and nut-free (see pages 7–9)*

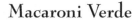

Macaroni Verde

*Fresh herbs, garlic, and lemon combine to make the
sauce for this zesty and flavorful pasta side dish.*

Preparation time: 10 minutes
Cooking time: 10 minutes

1 (8 ounce) package dairy-, egg-, and nut-free **elbow macaroni** (any
size)
2 cups firmly packed fresh basil leaves
½ cup firmly packed fresh parsley leaves (without stems)
½ cup olive oil
2 tablespoons freshly squeezed lemon juice
4 large cloves fresh garlic, peeled
1 tablespoon dairy- and egg-free **Dijon mustard**
½ teaspoon salt

Prepare macaroni according to the package directions; drain.

While macaroni is cooking, make sauce. Place remaining ingredients in
a food processor that has been fitted with the metal blade. Process until
basil, parsley, and garlic are all finely chopped and sauce is well mixed.

Place drained macaroni in a serving bowl. Pour sauce over macaroni
and toss to coat. Serve immediately.

Makes 4 servings (about 1 cup each).

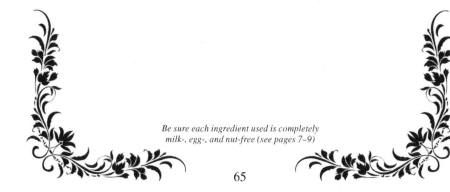

*Be sure each ingredient used is completely
milk-, egg-, and nut-free (see pages 7–9)*

Pasta with Roasted Vegetables

Team this up with melon balls and a loaf of dairy-, egg-, and nut-free French bread for a wonderful meatless supper.

Preparation time: 12 minutes
Cooking time: 20 minutes

1 (8 ounce) package dairy-, egg-, and nut-free **spiral pasta**
10 peeled baby-cut carrots
1 medium zucchini
¾ pound asparagus, preferably fairly thin
½ of a medium-size red bell pepper
¼ cup olive oil, divided use
1 tablespoon bottled **minced garlic**
salt and freshly ground black pepper, to taste
1 tablespoon dried thyme leaves
3 tablespoons **julienne-sliced sun-dried tomatoes packed in oil**,
    not drained

Preheat oven to 450 degrees F.

Prepare pasta according to the package directions; drain.

While the oven is heating and the water for cooking the pasta is boiling, prepare the vegetables. Cut carrots in quarters lengthwise. Trim ends off zucchini, cut zucchini in half lengthwise, and then cut into ¼-inch-thick slices. Remove and discard woody ends from asparagus and then cut asparagus into 1-inch-long pieces. Seed bell pepper and then cut into 1-inch-long by ¼-inch-wide strips.

Place prepared carrots, zucchini, asparagus, and bell pepper in a 9-inch by 13-inch baking dish. Add 2 tablespoons oil, garlic, salt, and pepper; mix well. Spread vegetables out evenly in the baking dish. Place in oven and cook, uncovered, for 10 minutes. Stir. Spread vegetables back out evenly in the dish and cook for an additional 10 minutes or until vegetables are tender when pierced with a fork.

Place cooked vegetables, drained pasta, thyme, sun-dried tomatoes, and remaining 2 tablespoons oil in a large serving bowl; mix well. Serve hot.

Makes 4 servings (about 1½ cups each).

*Be sure each ingredient used is completely
milk-, egg-, and nut-free (see pages 7–9)*

Rotini with Bread Crumbs

*This is a nice, "homey" pasta recipe, perfect for
your regular rotation of weeknight suppers.*

Preparation and cooking time: 25 minutes

1 (12 ounce) package dairy-, egg-, and nut-free **tri-colored rotini**
1 (8 ounce) package fresh button mushrooms
1 small slice dairy-, egg-, and nut-free **wheat bread**, torn into 4 pieces
2 tablespoons sherry wine
2 teaspoons bottled **minced garlic**
1 (14.5 ounce) can **diced and peeled tomatoes in tomato juice**,
     not drained
1 teaspoon dried basil leaves
1 teaspoon dried thyme leaves
½ teaspoon dried parsley leaves

Prepare pasta according to the package directions; drain.

While the pasta is cooking, prepare the rest of the recipe. Wash
mushrooms. Using a food processor that has been fitted with the
medium slicing disk, slice mushrooms; set aside. Replace slicing
disk with metal blade; use food processor to process the bread slice
into crumbs.

Heat a 12-inch skillet over high heat. Add bread crumbs. Cook, stirring
quite frequently, until lightly toasted, about 2 minutes. Remove toasted
bread crumbs from skillet and set aside.

Reduce heat to medium-high. Place sherry, garlic, and sliced
mushrooms in skillet. Sauté, stirring frequently, until mushrooms are
soft, about 2 minutes. Stir in tomatoes (with juice), basil, thyme, and
parsley. Cook just until heated through. Remove from heat.

Place drained pasta and cooked tomato mixture in a serving bowl;
mix. Serve hot, with toasted bread crumbs sprinkled over the top of
each serving.

Makes 6 servings (1¼ cups each).

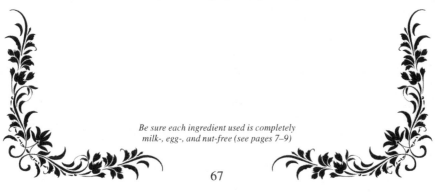

*Be sure each ingredient used is completely
milk-, egg-, and nut-free (see pages 7–9)*

Notes

Potatoes

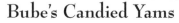

Bube's Candied Yams

Here is my grandmother's recipe for candied yams. There are two secrets to success with this recipe: start with yams that are, as my grandmother would say, "just the right size," and be sure to baste the yams every 15 minutes.

Preparation time: 15 minutes
Cooking time: 1 hour 45 minutes

4 yams, about 10 to 12 ounces each, each with a maximum diameter of about 2 to 2½ inches
1 tablespoon + 1 teaspoon dairy-free **margarine**
1 tablespoon + 1 teaspoon honey
2¼ cups pineapple juice (three 6 ounce cans)
¼ cup firmly packed pure cane dark brown sugar

Scrub yams and place in a single layer in an 8-quart pot; add enough water to just cover the yams. Cover the pot and bring to a boil over high heat. Reduce the heat to low and simmer for about 15 minutes, until the yams can be easily pierced with a fork. Drain yams in a colander and then cool in colander for 10 minutes.

Preheat oven to 350 degrees F.

Carefully peel yams. Slice each yam in half lengthwise. Place yam halves in a 9-inch by 13-inch baking dish. Place ½ teaspoon margarine on each yam, and then drizzle each yam with ½ teaspoon honey. Place the pineapple juice and brown sugar in a medium mixing bowl; mix well. Pour juice mixture over and around yams, being careful not to cause the margarine to fall off the yams. Bake, uncovered, for 1 hour 15 minutes, basting yams with the pineapple juice mixture from the baking dish every 15 minutes during the cooking time. Serve hot.

Makes 4 servings (1 yam each).

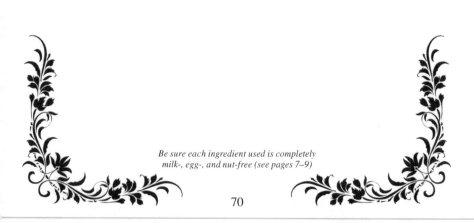

*Be sure each ingredient used is completely
milk-, egg-, and nut-free (see pages 7–9)*

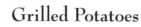

Grilled Potatoes

*Serve these potatoes, which are slightly hard on the outside
and tender in the middle, with grilled poultry or meat.*

Preparation time: 5 minutes
Cooking time: 15 minutes

2 pounds medium or large red new potatoes
3 tablespoons dairy-free **margarine**
2 tablespoons dairy- and egg-free **Dijon mustard**
1 tablespoon dried rosemary, crumbled

Heat gas grill.

Scrub potatoes and cut lengthwise into ⅜- to ½-inch-wide slices. Place margarine in a large microwave-safe bowl. Microwave on high until melted, about 30 seconds. Add mustard and rosemary; mix well. Add potato slices; mix well to coat.

Arrange prepared potato slices in a single layer on preheated grill. Cook for 7 minutes over high heat. Turn slices over and then cook for about 7 more minutes, until potatoes are tender when pierced with a fork. Serve hot.

Makes 4 servings.

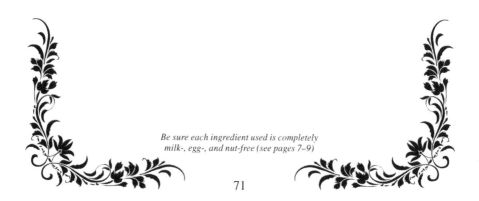

*Be sure each ingredient used is completely
milk-, egg-, and nut-free (see pages 7–9)*

Rosemary Red Potatoes

Here's a satisfying potato dish for a cold winter's night.

Preparation time: 6 minutes
Cooking time: 20 minutes

2 pounds red new potatoes
⅓ cup olive oil
1 tablespoon dairy- and egg-free **Dijon mustard**
1 tablespoon dried rosemary, crumbled
Salt, to taste

Scrub potatoes; cut into approximately 1-inch chunks. Place in a
3-quart pot and add enough water to just cover potatoes. Cover pot and
bring to a boil over high heat. Reduce heat to low and simmer, covered,
for 10 minutes or until potatoes are slightly tender when pierced with a
fork; drain.

While potatoes are cooking, make sauce. Place oil, mustard, rosemary,
and salt in a small bowl; mix well with a fork or small wire whisk.

Place cooked, drained potatoes and sauce in a serving bowl; gently mix
until potatoes are coated with sauce. Serve hot.

Makes 6 servings (about 1 cup each).

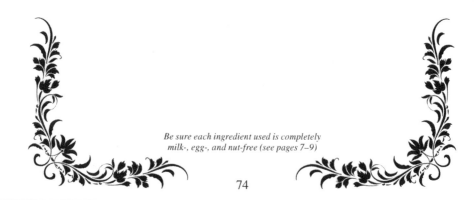

*Be sure each ingredient used is completely
milk-, egg-, and nut-free (see pages 7–9)*

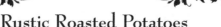

Rustic Roasted Potatoes

This goes well with meatloaf or roasted chicken.

Preparation time: 10 minutes
Cooking time: 1 hour

2 pounds russet potatoes
1 medium brown onion
1 cup peeled baby-cut carrots
⅓ cup olive oil
2 teaspoons freshly squeezed lemon juice
2 teaspoons bottled **minced garlic**
2 teaspoons dried rosemary, crumbled
1 teaspoon dried thyme leaves
1 teaspoon salt
½ teaspoon black pepper

Heat oven to 400 degrees F.

Scrub potatoes and cut into approximately ½-inch chunks. Peel and chop onion. Slice carrots in half lengthwise.

Place prepared vegetables in a 9-inch by 13-inch baking dish. Place remaining ingredients in a measuring cup; mix well. Pour olive oil mixture over vegetables; mix well. Spread vegetables out evenly in pan.

Bake, uncovered, for about 1 hour, stirring once during cooking time, until potatoes feel tender when pierced with a fork. Serve hot.

Makes 6 servings (about 1¼ cups each).

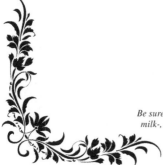

*Be sure each ingredient used is completely
milk-, egg-, and nut-free (see pages 7–9)*

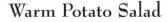

Warm Potato Salad

While this is probably not a good choice to serve to toddlers and young children, teenagers and adults give it high marks!

Preparation time: 20 minutes
Cooking time: 25 minutes
Sitting time: 10 minutes

2 pounds red new potatoes
5 green onions (scallions)
¼ cup + 1 tablespoon olive oil, divided use
2 tablespoons + 2 teaspoons **white wine vinegar**
1½ teaspoons bottled **minced garlic**
1½ teaspoons **Worcestershire sauce**
2 tablespoons sherry wine
salt and pepper, to taste

Scrub potatoes and place in a single layer in a 4-quart pot; add enough water to cover potatoes by about ½ inch. Cover and bring to a boil over high heat. Reduce heat to low and simmer, covered, for about 25 minutes or until the potatoes can be easily pierced with a fork; drain.

While potatoes are cooking, prepare remaining ingredients. Mince green onions, including the green tops; set aside. To make dressing place ¼ cup olive oil, vinegar, garlic, and Worcestershire sauce in a small bowl or measuring cup; mix well and set aside.

Cut cooked and drained potatoes into quarters or eighths (depending on size) and place in a large serving bowl. Add minced green onions, remaining 1 tablespoon olive oil, sherry, salt, and pepper; gently toss to coat. Allow to sit 10 minutes. Pour dressing over potato mixture and toss lightly; serve.

Makes 5 servings (1 cup each).

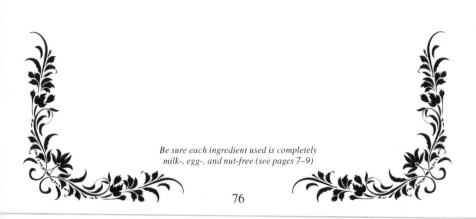

Be sure each ingredient used is completely milk-, egg-, and nut-free (see pages 7–9)

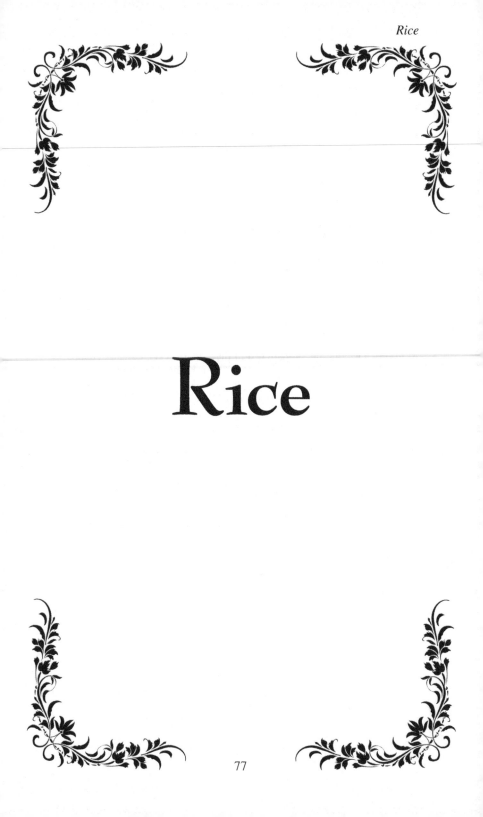

Rice

Fruity Rice

Apples and dried cranberries sweeten this rice dish.

Preparation time: 8 minutes
Cooking time: 20 minutes

2 cups water
1 cup long-grain **white rice**
1 small red apple
½ of a small brown onion
1 tablespoon dairy-free **margarine**
¼ cup **sweetened dried cranberries**
1 tablespoon firmly packed pure cane brown sugar
⅛ teaspoon ground allspice
⅛ teaspoon ground nutmeg

Place water in a 2-quart pot; cover and bring to a boil over high heat. Stir in rice. Reduce heat to low and cook, covered, for 18 minutes or until all water has been absorbed.

While rice is cooking, prepare rest of ingredients. Peel, core, and chop apple. Peel and chop onion; you should have ½ cup. Melt margarine in 10- or 12-inch skillet over medium-high heat. Add chopped apple and onion and cook, stirring frequently, for approximately 5 minutes or until onions are soft. Remove skillet from heat and stir in dried cranberries, brown sugar, allspice, and nutmeg; set aside.

When rice is cooked remove from heat and add prepared fruit mixture; mix well. Serve hot.

Makes 5 servings (about ¾ cup each).

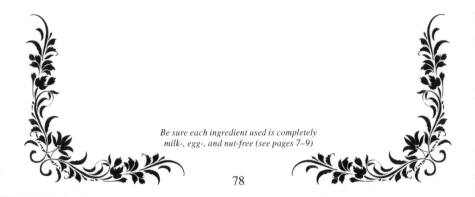

*Be sure each ingredient used is completely
milk-, egg-, and nut-free (see pages 7–9)*

Have It Your Way Rice

Is your family tired of plain rice? Or, more likely, are some members of your family tired of plain rice while others cringe at the thought of anything "fancy"? Now you can make everyone happy.

Next time you make rice create a special "rice bar" (similar to a baked potato or taco bar). Put out a big bowl of cooked rice and a whole variety of potential "add-ins," and let everyone make their own rice creation. Here are some add-in ideas to get you started...

Asian
dairy-free **soy sauce**, bottled **minced ginger**, and fresh minced chives or green onions

Exotic
Chinese 5-Spice Powder

Indian
curry powder

Italian
dried basil leaves, garlic powder, and **lemon pepper**

Mexican
salsa or **picante sauce**

Peach Pie
peach jam (melted in microwave oven), ground nutmeg

Spicy
Tabasco sauce

Sugar & Spice
raisins, sugar, and ground cinnamon

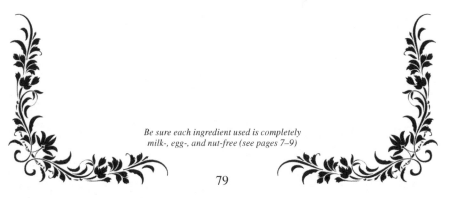

Be sure each ingredient used is completely milk-, egg-, and nut-free (see pages 7–9)

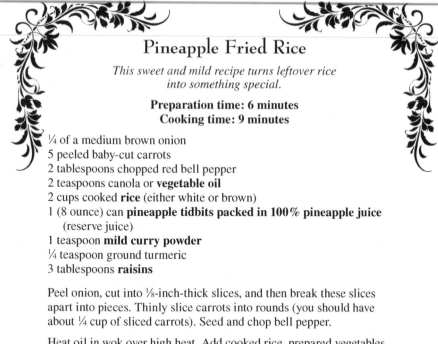

Pineapple Fried Rice

This sweet and mild recipe turns leftover rice into something special.

Preparation time: 6 minutes
Cooking time: 9 minutes

¼ of a medium brown onion
5 peeled baby-cut carrots
2 tablespoons chopped red bell pepper
2 teaspoons canola or **vegetable oil**
2 cups cooked **rice** (either white or brown)
1 (8 ounce) can **pineapple tidbits packed in 100% pineapple juice**
  (reserve juice)
1 teaspoon **mild curry powder**
¼ teaspoon ground turmeric
3 tablespoons **raisins**

Peel onion, cut into ⅛-inch-thick slices, and then break these slices apart into pieces. Thinly slice carrots into rounds (you should have about ¼ cup of sliced carrots). Seed and chop bell pepper.

Heat oil in wok over high heat. Add cooked rice, prepared vegetables, ⅓ cup pineapple juice from the canned pineapple, curry powder, and turmeric. Stir-fry about 8 to 9 minutes or until onions are soft, stirring often. Add raisins and drained pineapple; cook for about 30 seconds, just until raisins and pineapple are warm. Serve immediately.

Makes 4 servings (¾ cup each).

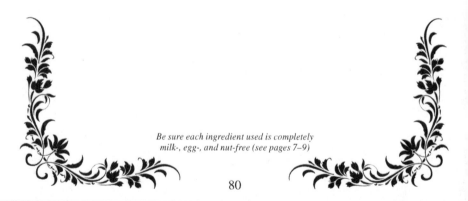

*Be sure each ingredient used is completely
milk-, egg-, and nut-free (see pages 7–9)*

Rice Jubilee

This colorful rice dish is a nice change of pace.

Preparation time: 7 minutes
Cooking time: 22 minutes

2 cups water
1 cup long-grain **white rice**
1 cup packaged shredded carrots
1 (8 ounce) can **pineapple tidbits packed in 100% pineapple juice**,
  not drained
1 tablespoon olive oil
1 tablespoon dairy-free **low-sodium soy sauce**
1 teaspoon bottled **minced ginger**
½ teaspoon dried thyme leaves
½ teaspoon **Chinese 5-Spice Powder**
salt and freshly ground black pepper, to taste
1 green onion (scallion)
5 **dried apricot halves**
1 (8.5 ounce) can "no salt added" **whole kernel corn**, drained

Place water in a 3-quart pot; cover and bring to a boil over high heat.
Stir in rice and shredded carrots. Reduce heat to low and cook, covered,
for 18 minutes or until all liquid has been absorbed. Remove from heat
and let sit for 2 minutes, covered.

While rice and carrots are cooking, prepare rest of ingredients. To
make dressing, place 3 tablespoons of the pineapple juice from the
canned pineapple, oil, soy sauce, ginger, thyme, Chinese 5-Spice
Powder, salt, and pepper in a small bowl; mix well. Finely chop green
onion and chop apricot halves. Drain corn and pineapple.

Place cooked rice, dressing, green onions, dried apricots, corn, and
pineapple in a serving bowl; mix well. Serve hot.

Makes 6 servings (about ¾ cup each).

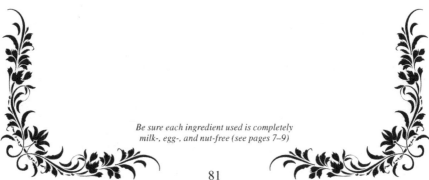

*Be sure each ingredient used is completely
milk-, egg-, and nut-free (see pages 7–9)*

Rice Pilaf

Just like they serve at restaurants!

Preparation time: 10 minutes
Cooking time: 18 minutes

½ of a small brown onion
1 tablespoon dairy-free **margarine**
⅓ cup dairy-, egg-, and nut-free **cut fideo pasta** (this pasta comes
   already broken into small pieces)
1 (14.5 ounce) can dairy- and egg-free **fat-free reduced-sodium
   chicken broth** (1¼ cups broth)
¼ cup water
1 cup long-grain **white rice**
salt and pepper to taste

Peel and chop onion; you should have ½ cup. Melt margarine in a
2-quart saucepan over medium-high heat. Add chopped onion and
sauté over high heat for 1 minute, stirring frequently. Add pasta and
sauté for another 1 to 2 minutes, stirring frequently, until pasta is
slightly browned.

Add chicken broth and water to saucepan; cover and bring to a boil over
high heat. Reduce heat to low and stir in rice, salt, and pepper. Cook,
covered, for 18 minutes or until all liquid has been absorbed. Serve hot.

Makes 4 servings (about ¾ cup each).

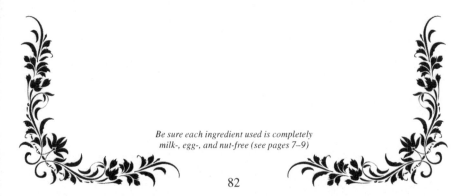

*Be sure each ingredient used is completely
milk-, egg-, and nut-free (see pages 7–9)*

Tomato Rice

Cook this up for the tomato lovers in your household.

Preparation time: 10 minutes
Cooking time: 25 minutes

¼ of a small brown onion
1 tablespoon dairy-free **margarine**
1 (14½ ounce) can **diced and peeled tomatoes in tomato juice**,
    not drained
1 (5.5 ounce) can **low-sodium 100% vegetable juice** (about ⅔ cup)
1 cup water
1 cup long-grain **white rice**

Peel and chop onion; you should have ¼ cup. Heat margarine in
a 3-quart pot over high heat. Add chopped onions and sauté for 2
minutes, stirring constantly. Add tomatoes, vegetable juice, and water.
Cover and bring to a boil over high heat. Stir in rice. Reduce heat to low
and simmer, covered, for 20 minutes or until rice is tender and most
(but not quite all) of the liquid has been absorbed. Serve hot.

Makes 5 servings (¾ cup each).

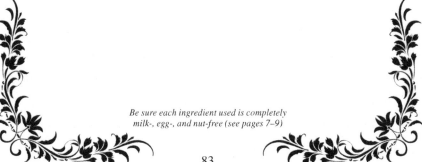

*Be sure each ingredient used is completely
milk-, egg-, and nut-free (see pages 7–9)*

Notes

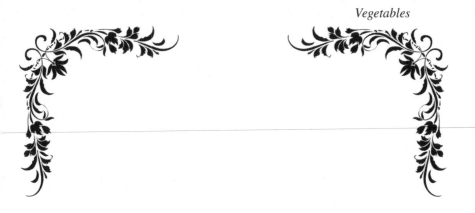

Vegetables

Candied Carrots

My grandmother used to make carrots this way – as sweet as candy.

Preparation time: 5 minutes
Cooking time: 40 minutes

1 (1 pound) bag peeled baby-cut carrots or 1 pound carrots, peeled
¼ cup honey
¼ cup firmly packed pure cane dark brown sugar

Using a food processor that has been fitted with the slicing disk, slice carrots into rounds. Place sliced carrots into a 2-quart saucepan and add just enough water so that the carrots are barely covered. Cover and bring to a boil over high heat. Reduce heat to low and simmer, covered, until carrots are tender when pierced with a fork, about 10 minutes.

Drain carrots, reserving ¼ cup of the cooking liquid. Place cooked carrots, reserved cooking liquid, honey, and brown sugar in the saucepan; stir gently. Return to a boil over high heat and then reduce heat to low and simmer, covered, for 15 minutes, stirring occasionally. Using a slotted spoon, transfer cooked carrots to a serving dish. Serve hot.

Makes 4 servings (over ½ cup each).

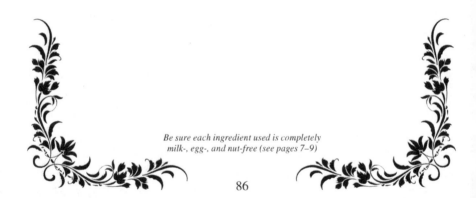

*Be sure each ingredient used is completely
milk-, egg-, and nut-free (see pages 7–9)*

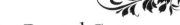

Dilled Pan-Roasted Carrots

*If you like the taste of fresh dill, give this
refreshingly different carrot dish a try.*

**Preparation time: 4 minutes
Cooking time: 17 to 20 minutes**

1 (1 pound) bag peeled baby-cut carrots, preferably not too thick
1 tablespoon olive oil
½ of a small brown onion
1 tablespoon firmly packed fresh dill leaves
2 tablespoons freshly squeezed lemon juice

Place carrots in a 12-inch skillet. Add oil; mix well. Spread carrots
out so that they form a single layer in the skillet. Peel and finely chop
onion and then sprinkle over the carrots. Cover skillet and cook over
medium-low heat for 10 minutes; stir. Chop dill leaves. Add chopped
dill and lemon juice to skillet; stir. Cover and cook an additional 7 to
10 minutes, until carrots are slightly tender when pierced with a fork.
Serve hot.

Makes 2½ servings (¾ cup each).

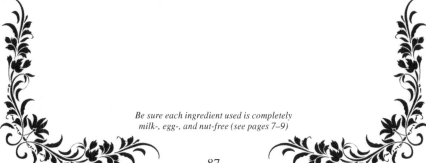

*Be sure each ingredient used is completely
milk-, egg-, and nut-free (see pages 7–9)*

Grated Zucchini Sauté

This makes a light and summery vegetable side dish.

Preparation time: 3 minutes
Cooking time: 10 minutes

½ cup firmly packed fresh basil leaves
1½ pounds zucchini (about 3 medium zucchini)
1 tablespoon dairy-free **margarine**
1 teaspoon dairy- and egg-free **Dijon mustard**
freshly ground black pepper to taste
salt to taste (optional)

Fit a food processor with the metal blade. Turn on the food processor and drop the basil through the feeding tube while the machine is running. Turn off the food processor and replace the metal blade with the grating disk. Trim ends off zucchini and then use the food processor to grate the zucchini.

Melt margarine in a 12-inch skillet over medium heat. Add mustard; mix well. Add prepared zucchini, basil, pepper, and (optional) salt. Cook, stirring frequently, for about 8 minutes. Serve hot.

Makes 4 servings.

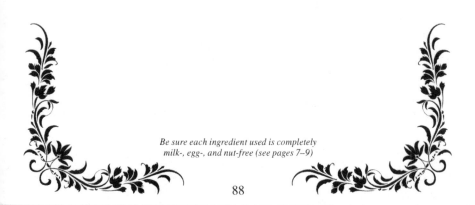

*Be sure each ingredient used is completely
milk-, egg-, and nut-free (see pages 7–9)*

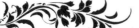

Grilled Asparagus with Rosemary

Grilling can take asparagus from simple to sublime.
For best results, use thin asparagus spears.

Preparation time: 3 minutes
Cooking time: 5 minutes

1 pound fresh asparagus, preferably fairly thin
1 tablespoon olive oil
1½ teaspoons dried rosemary, crumbled
salt and pepper, to taste

Preheat barbecue.

While barbecue is heating, remove and discard woody ends from asparagus. Place asparagus in shallow dish and toss with olive oil, rosemary, salt, and pepper.

Carefully place the asparagus on the heated grill, perpendicular to the grid. Grill, turning occasionally, until the asparagus is tender, about 3 to 5 minutes (depending on the thickness of the asparagus spears). Serve immediately.

Makes 4 servings.

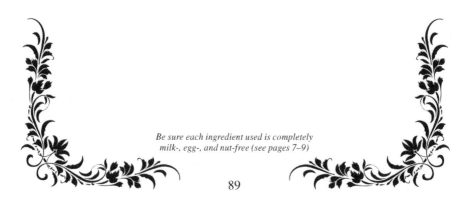

Be sure each ingredient used is completely
milk-, egg-, and nut-free (see pages 7–9)

89

What Else is to Eat?

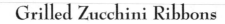

Grilled Zucchini Ribbons

This is one of my favorite ways to prepare zucchini.

Preparation time: 6 minutes
Cooking time: 6 to 8 minutes

1½ pounds zucchini (about 3 medium zucchini)
⅓ cup olive oil
1 teaspoon bottled **minced garlic**

Preheat barbecue.

Trim ends off zucchini and then slice zucchini lengthwise into ¼-inch-thick slices; place on a cookie sheet. Place oil and garlic in a small bowl or measuring cup; mix well. Brush oil mixture onto both sides of zucchini slices.

Remove zucchini slices from cookie sheet and place on the heated grill. Cook 2 to 3 minutes per side or until done. Serve immediately.

Makes 4 servings.

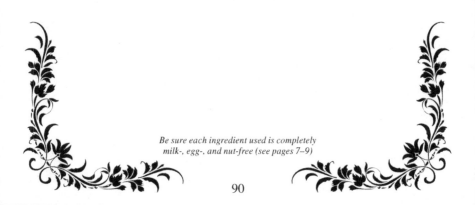

*Be sure each ingredient used is completely
milk-, egg-, and nut-free (see pages 7–9)*

Italian Vegetable Sauté

This makes an appealingly colorful presentation.

Preparation time: 5 minutes
Cooking time: 10 minutes

1 medium zucchini
1 medium yellow crookneck squash
½ of a small red bell pepper
½ of a small brown onion, peeled
1 tablespoon olive oil
⅓ cup **julienne-sliced sun-dried tomatoes packed in olive oil,**
   not drained
1 tablespoon dried basil leaves
1 teaspoon bottled **minced garlic**
freshly ground black pepper, to taste

Trim ends off zucchini and yellow squash and then slice into ¼-inch-thick rounds. Seed bell pepper and cut into ¼-inch-wide by 1½-inch-long strips. Cut onion in half and then cut into ¼-inch-thick slices.

Heat olive oil in a 12-inch skillet over medium-high heat. Add the prepared vegetables, sun-dried tomatoes, basil, garlic, and pepper. Sauté, stirring frequently, until vegetables are slightly soft, about 7 minutes. Serve hot.

Makes 4 servings (¾ cup each).

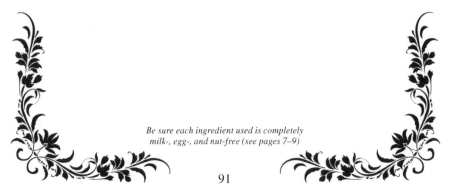

Be sure each ingredient used is completely
milk-, egg-, and nut-free (see pages 7–9)

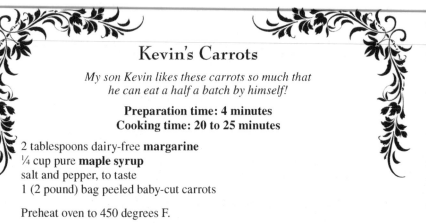

Kevin's Carrots

*My son Kevin likes these carrots so much that
he can eat a half a batch by himself!*

Preparation time: 4 minutes
Cooking time: 20 to 25 minutes

2 tablespoons dairy-free **margarine**
¼ cup pure **maple syrup**
salt and pepper, to taste
1 (2 pound) bag peeled baby-cut carrots

Preheat oven to 450 degrees F.

Place margarine in a microwave-safe bowl or measuring cup;
microwave on high until melted. Stir in maple syrup, salt, and pepper.

Place carrots in a 9-inch by 13-inch baking pan. Pour margarine/maple
syrup mixture over carrots. Mix well to coat and then spread out evenly
in pan.

Bake, uncovered, for 10 minutes. Stir carrots, spread back out evenly in
pan, and then bake for an additional 10 to 15 minutes, until carrots feel
tender when pierced with a fork. Serve hot.

Makes 6 servings (about ¾ cup each).

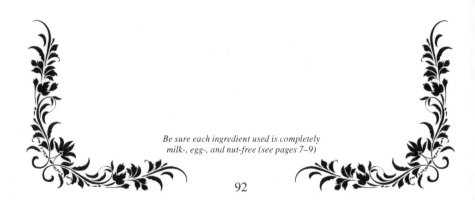

*Be sure each ingredient used is completely
milk-, egg-, and nut-free (see pages 7–9)*

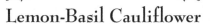

Lemon-Basil Cauliflower

This quick and easy dish is equally delicious served hot or cold.

Preparation time: 10 minutes
Cooking time: 15 minutes

1 medium-size head fresh cauliflower
3 tablespoons freshly squeezed lemon juice
1 tablespoon olive oil
1 tablespoon chopped fresh basil leaves or 2 teaspoons dried
   basil leaves
1 teaspoon dairy- and egg-free **Dijon mustard**
1 teaspoon bottled **minced garlic**
salt and pepper, to taste

Wash cauliflower; cut into bite-size florets.

Place prepared cauliflower in a 3-quart pot. Add just enough water to cover the cauliflower. Bring to a boil over high heat. Reduce heat to low and simmer, covered, 5 minutes, until cauliflower is tender when pierced with a fork. Drain and place in serving bowl.

While cauliflower is cooking, make dressing. Place all other ingredients in a small bowl; mix well.

Pour dressing over drained, cooked cauliflower; mix well. Serve hot, or refrigerate and serve cold as a salad.

Makes 6 servings (about ¾ cup each).

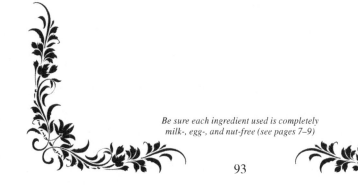

Be sure each ingredient used is completely
milk-, egg-, and nut-free (see pages 7–9)

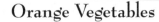

Orange Vegetables

This bright orange-colored side dish really perks up the dinner plate!

Preparation time: 5 minutes
Cooking time: 25 minutes

10 **dried apricot halves**
1 (14 ounce) yam, maximum 2½ inches diameter at its thickest part
2 tablespoons dairy-free **margarine**
1 cup peeled baby-cut carrots
½ cup apple juice
½ cup **orange juice**
1 tablespoon freshly-grated orange peel
½ teaspoon ground cinnamon

Slice dried apricot pieces into thirds; set aside. Peel yam, slice in half lengthwise, and then slice into ¼-inch-thick slices.

Melt margarine in a 12-inch skillet over medium-high heat. Add carrots and sliced yams; cook over medium-high heat for 3 minutes, stirring frequently. Stir in dried apricots, apple juice, orange juice, grated orange peel, and cinnamon. Bring to a boil over high heat. Reduce heat to low, stir, and then simmer for 15 minutes, covered. Uncover skillet and cook for an additional 5 minutes, until yams and carrots are tender when pierced with a fork. Using a slotted spoon, remove cooked vegetables from skillet and place in a serving dish. Serve hot.

Makes 4 servings (about ¾ cup each).

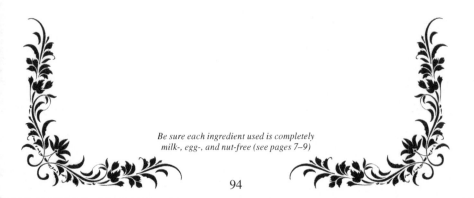

Be sure each ingredient used is completely milk-, egg-, and nut-free (see pages 7–9)

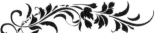

Quick and Easy Sautéed Asparagus

*One of my boys (who does not particularly care for asparagus)
declared that this is "about as good as asparagus gets." Those
who actually like asparagus give it even higher marks!*

**Preparation time: 4 minutes
Cooking time: 3 to 6 minutes**

1 pound fresh asparagus
1 tablespoon dairy-free **low-sodium soy sauce**
1 tablespoon **red wine vinegar**
½ teaspoon bottled **minced garlic**
½ teaspoon bottled **minced ginger**
1 tablespoon canola or **vegetable oil**

Remove and discard woody ends from asparagus, and then slice
asparagus diagonally into 2-inch-long pieces

Place soy sauce, vinegar, garlic, and ginger in a small bowl; mix well.

Heat oil in a 12-inch skillet over high heat. Add prepared asparagus and
sauce. Sauté 3 to 6 minutes (depending on the thickness of the asparagus
spears), until easily pierced with a fork. Serve hot.

Makes 4 servings (about ¾ cup each).

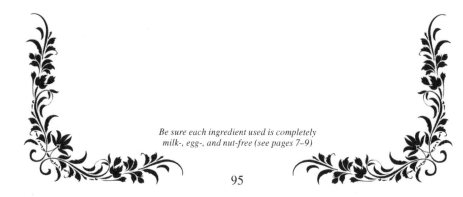

*Be sure each ingredient used is completely
milk-, egg-, and nut-free (see pages 7–9)*

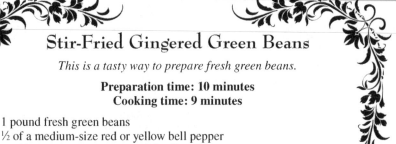

Stir-Fried Gingered Green Beans

This is a tasty way to prepare fresh green beans.

Preparation time: 10 minutes
Cooking time: 9 minutes

1 pound fresh green beans
½ of a medium-size red or yellow bell pepper
1 tablespoon canola or **vegetable oil**
¼ cup dairy-free **low-sodium soy sauce**
2 teaspoons bottled **minced ginger**
freshly ground black pepper, to taste

Wash and trim green beans; cut into 2-inch-long pieces. Seed and chop bell pepper.

Heat oil in wok over high heat. Add green beans, chopped bell pepper, soy sauce, ginger, and pepper. Stir-fry until green beans are tender-crisp, stirring frequently, about 7 minutes. Serve hot.

Makes 4 large servings (1 cup each).

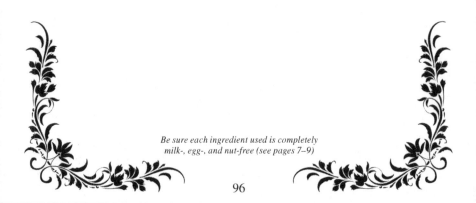

*Be sure each ingredient used is completely
milk-, egg-, and nut-free (see pages 7–9)*

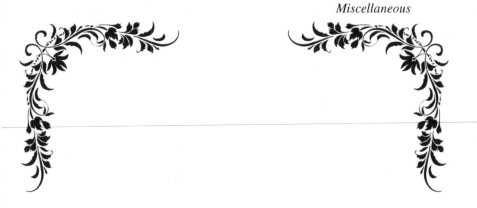

Miscellaneous

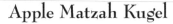

Apple Matzah Kugel

*Looking for something to serve during Passover? Try this
sweet dish with a traditional "matzah kugel" texture.*

Preparation time: 15 minutes
Cooking time: 30 minutes
Cooling time: 15 minutes

4 **matzahs**
¼ cup canola or **vegetable oil**
¼ cup pure cane sugar
¼ cup **apple sauce**
1 teaspoon ground cinnamon
2 medium red apples
½ cup **raisins**

Preheat oven to 450 degrees F. Using dairy-free **vegetable shortening**, grease an 8-inch square baking pan or glass baking dish; set aside.

Break matzah into pieces and place in a medium bowl. Cover with cold water; set aside.

Place oil, sugar, apple sauce, and cinnamon in a large mixing bowl; mix well. Peel and core apples. Grate apples using a food processor that has been fitted with the grating disk.

Place matzah in a colander to drain, pushing down with the back of a spoon to squeeze the water out. Add grated apples, drained matzah, and raisins to oil mixture in bowl; mix well. Spoon into prepared baking pan. Bake for about 30 minutes, until top is lightly browned and apples are cooked through. Cool for at least 15 minutes before serving, to give the kugel a chance to set. Cut into 9 pieces. Serve warm.

Makes 9 servings (approximately 2½ inches by 2½ inches each).

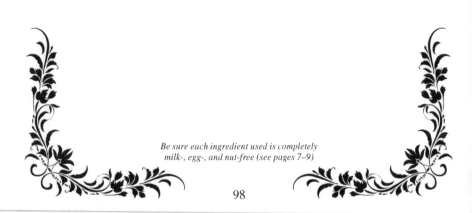

*Be sure each ingredient used is completely
milk-, egg-, and nut-free (see pages 7–9)*

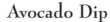

Avocado Dip

I really enjoy this mild version of guacamole. Serve it with tortilla chips at your next party, or whip up a batch for an afternoon snack.

Preparation time: 8 to 10 minutes

4 very ripe avocados
½ of a medium tomato
1 green onion (scallion)
1 teaspoon freshly squeezed lemon juice
¼ teaspoon garlic powder
salt and pepper, to taste

Cut avocadoes in half and remove pits. Using a spoon, scoop out the avocado flesh and put it in a medium mixing bowl. Using a fork or potato masher, mash the avocados until no large lumps remain.

Seed and finely chop the tomato (you should have about ¼ cup chopped tomato). Thinly slice the green onion (including the green top).

Add prepared tomato and green onion, lemon juice, garlic powder, salt, and pepper to mashed avocado; mix well. Serve cold or at room temperature. Refrigerate any leftovers.

Makes about 1½ cups dip.

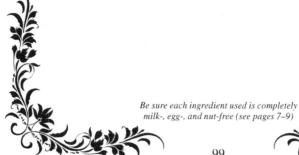

*Be sure each ingredient used is completely
milk-, egg-, and nut-free (see pages 7–9)*

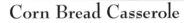

Corn Bread Casserole

If you like corn bread, you'll love this casserole. Serve it up with a
salad or green vegetable for supper, bring it to your next potluck
dinner, or enjoy it as a nice change-of-pace brunch dish.

Preparation time: 20 to 25 minutes
Cooking time: 45 minutes

½ cup chopped brown onion
½ cup finely chopped red or green bell pepper
¼ cup finely chopped celery
1 pound lean ground beef
½ teaspoon **seasoned salt**
½ teaspoon garlic powder
freshly ground black pepper, to taste
1 (14¾ ounce) can **cream-style corn**
1 cup **yellow cornmeal**
1 cup **all-purpose flour**
¼ cup pure cane sugar
¾ cup **vanilla-flavored soy milk** or **rice milk**
¼ cup canola or **vegetable oil**, plus extra for greasing pan
2 tablespoons canola or **vegetable oil**, 2 tablespoons water, and
   2 teaspoons **baking powder**, mixed together
1 teaspoon **baking soda**

Preheat oven to 375 degrees F. Using canola or **vegetable oil**, grease a
9-inch by 13-inch baking pan.

Chop vegetables. Place chopped vegetables, ground beef, seasoned salt,
garlic powder, and pepper in a 12-inch skillet. Cook over medium-high
heat, stirring frequently and breaking meat up into small pieces as
you stir, until beef is completely cooked through (with no pink or red
showing); drain.

Place remaining ingredients in a large mixing bowl; mix well. Stir in
cooked and drained meat mixture. Pour evenly into prepared baking
pan. Bake for about 45 minutes, until the top is somewhat browned and
a toothpick inserted into the center of the casserole comes out clean.
Serve hot.

Makes 6 main-dish servings
(approximately 3 inches by 4¼ inches each).

Be sure each ingredient used is completely
milk-, egg-, and nut-free (see pages 7–9)

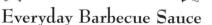

Everyday Barbecue Sauce

*Use this quickly-assembled condiment as an
alternative to bottled barbecue sauce.*

Preparation time: 5 minutes

1 (6 ounce) can **tomato paste**
¼ cup unsulfured **molasses**
¼ cup **apple cider vinegar**
¼ cup water
2 teaspoons dried minced onion
1 teaspoon paprika
1 teaspoon ground mustard powder
1 teaspoon ground oregano
1 teaspoon ground thyme
1 teaspoon bottled **minced garlic**
½ teaspoon black pepper

Place all ingredients in a medium bowl; stir.

Makes 1⅓ cups (enough to baste 2½ pounds of cut-up chicken pieces).

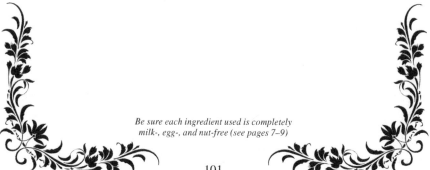

*Be sure each ingredient used is completely
milk-, egg-, and nut-free (see pages 7–9)*

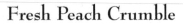

Fresh Peach Crumble

Turn fresh peaches into a mouth-watering dessert!

Preparation time: 10 minutes
Cooking time: 20 to 25 minutes

2 pounds firm fresh peaches
2 tablespoons pure cane sugar, divided use
⅓ cup quick-cooking oats
¼ cup + 1 tablespoon **all-purpose flour**
3 tablespoons chilled dairy-free **margarine**
2 tablespoons firmly packed pure cane dark brown sugar

Preheat oven to 375 degrees F.

Using a vegetable peeler, peel peaches. Cut peaches in half, remove pits, and then cut each half into about 7 slices. Place sliced peaches in a medium mixing bowl and gently toss with 1 tablespoon sugar.

Place remaining ingredients in a food processor that has been fitted with the metal blade; quickly process using a pulsing motion until mixture starts to form clumps. Spread peaches out evenly in a 9-inch pie pan or a 9-inch round cake pan. Sprinkle crumble mixture evenly over peaches.

Bake for 20 to 25 minutes, until crumble is golden brown. Cool 10 minutes and then serve warm.

Makes 4 large servings.

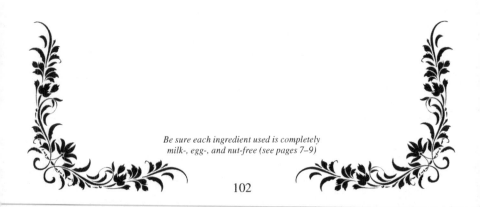

*Be sure each ingredient used is completely
milk-, egg-, and nut-free (see pages 7–9)*

Sun-Dried Tomato Spread

*This is an incredibly easy-to-make spread that
always gets rave reviews at parties.*

Preparation time: 3 minutes

1 (8½ ounce) jar **sun-dried tomatoes packed in oil**, room
    temperature, not drained
1 teaspoon bottled **minced garlic**
¼ cup firmly packed fresh basil leaves
¼ cup firmly packed fresh parsley leaves

Place all ingredients in a food processor that has been fitted with the
metal blade. Process until pureed and well blended. Serve either cold
or at room temperature, with dairy-, egg-, and nut-free crackers (it goes
especially well with "water crackers").

Makes 1 cup of spread.

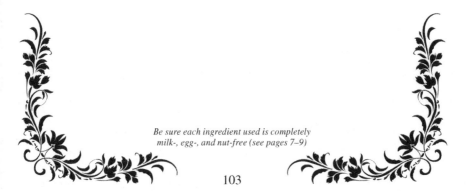

*Be sure each ingredient used is completely
milk-, egg-, and nut-free (see pages 7–9)*

Veggie Wraps

Tired of sandwiches? Try these wraps for a nice vegetarian lunch.

Preparation time: 8 to 10 minutes

2 teaspoons olive oil
2 teaspoons **white wine vinegar**
¼ teaspoon cumin
salt and pepper to taste
1 medium avocado, ripe
¼ of a medium cucumber
1 small tomato
⅓ cup shredded iceberg lettuce
4 (8-inch-diameter) **flour tortillas**, room temperature
2 tablespoons **raisins**

Place oil, vinegar, cumin, salt, and pepper in a small bowl or measuring cup; mix well and then set aside.

Peel and pit avocado; slice. Peel and chop cucumber. Cut tomato into thin slices and then cut each slice in thirds. Shred lettuce.

Place tortillas on a flat surface. Place dressing, prepared vegetables, and raisins in a medium mixing bowl; toss gently. Divide vegetable mixture and raisins evenly between the 4 tortillas, placing the ingredients on the top middle section of each tortilla. Fold bottom half of each tortilla up and over filling. Fold sides of each tortilla inwards. Serve.

Makes 4 servings (1 wrap each).

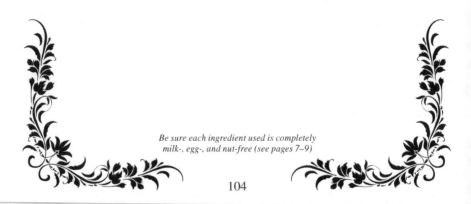

*Be sure each ingredient used is completely
milk-, egg-, and nut-free (see pages 7–9)*

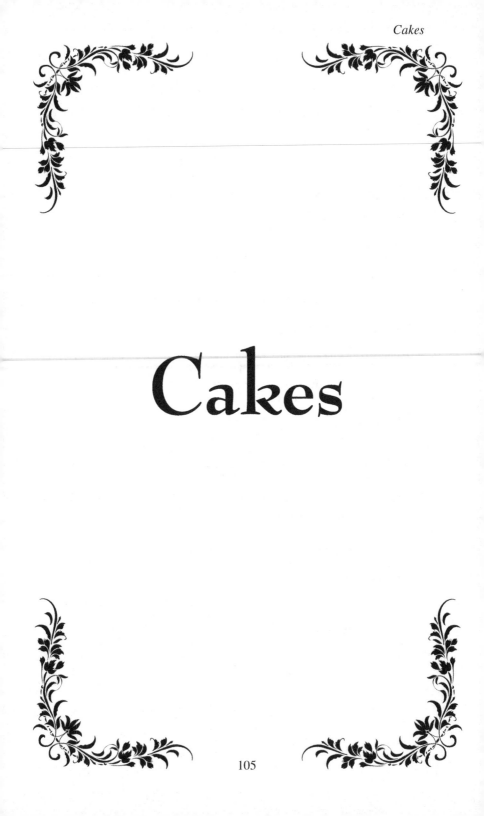

Cakes

Cherry Streusel Cake

*This cake forms 3 "layers" as it cooks – a soft layer
of cherries on the bottom, the cake in the middle, and
a sweet crunchy streusel on top. Delicious!*

Preparation time: 12 minutes
Cooking time: 30 to 35 minutes

Streusel

¼ cup **all-purpose flour**
¼ cup pure cane sugar
½ teaspoon ground cinnamon
1½ tablespoons dairy-free **margarine**, chilled

Cake

1 (16.5 ounce) can **pitted dark sweet bing cherries in heavy syrup**,
    not drained
1½ cups **all-purpose flour**
1 cup pure cane sugar
1 (6 ounce) can pineapple juice (¾ cup juice)
2 tablespoons canola or **vegetable oil**, 2 tablespoons water, and
    2 teaspoons **baking powder**, mixed together
2 tablespoons canola or **vegetable oil**
2 teaspoons **baking soda**
1 teaspoon **pure vanilla extract**

Preheat oven to 400 degrees F. Using dairy-free **vegetable
shortening**, grease a 10-inch quiche dish.

Place ¼ cup flour, ¼ cup sugar, and ½ teaspoon cinnamon in a small
bowl; mix well. Using a pastry blender cut in the margarine until
mixture resembles coarse crumbs; set aside.

Drain cherries, reserving ⅓ cup syrup. Place the reserved cherry syrup
and all remaining ingredients except the cherries in a large mixing
bowl; mix well with a wire whisk. Using a rubber spatula, gently fold in
the drained cherries.

Pour cake batter evenly into prepared quiche dish. Spoon streusel
mixture evenly on top of batter. Bake for 30 to 35 minutes or until
streusel is lightly browned and a toothpick inserted into the center of
the cake comes out clean. Cool 20 minutes before serving. Refrigerate
any leftovers.

Makes 8 servings.

*Be sure each ingredient used is completely
milk-, egg-, and nut-free (see pages 7–9)*

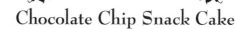

Chocolate Chip Snack Cake

*A wonderful "any time" cake, perfect for when you
don't want a traditional frosted layer cake.*

Preparation time: 25 minutes
Cooking time: 25 to 30 minutes

Cake

1½ cups **all-purpose flour**
⅔ cup pure cane sugar
1 cup water
⅓ cup canola or **vegetable oil**
2 tablespoons **white distilled vinegar**
2 teaspoons **baking powder**
2 teaspoons **pure vanilla extract**
⅔ cup dairy- and nut-free **semi-sweet chocolate chips**, divided use

Topping

¼ cup pure cane sugar
3 tablespoons dairy-free **margarine**, chilled, cut into pieces
3 tablespoons **all-purpose flour**
3 tablespoons dairy-free unsweetened **cocoa powder**

Preheat oven to 375 degrees F. Using dairy-free **vegetable shortening**,
grease and then flour an 8-inch square baking pan.

To make cake batter, place 1½ cups flour, ⅔ cup sugar, water, oil,
vinegar, baking powder, and vanilla in a large mixing bowl; mix well
with a wire whisk. Pour 1½ cups of batter evenly into prepared pan.
Bake for 5 minutes. Meanwhile, place topping ingredients in a small
bowl. Using a pastry blender, blend until well mixed and mixture
begins to form small clumps; set aside.

Remove cake from oven after it has baked for 5 minutes. Sprinkle ⅓ cup
chocolate chips evenly over the cake. Carefully spoon remaining batter
over chocolate chips. Sprinkle remaining ⅓ cup chocolate chips evenly
over batter. Bake for an additional 5 minutes.

Remove cake from oven again. Sprinkle topping mixture evenly over
cake. Return cake to oven and cook for an additional 25 to 30 minutes,
until a toothpick inserted into the center of the cake (but not into a
melted chocolate chip) comes out clean. Cool completely and then cut
into 16 pieces before serving.

Makes 16 small servings (2 inches by 2 inches each).

*Be sure each ingredient used is completely
milk-, egg-, and nut-free (see pages 7–9)*

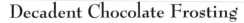

Decadent Chocolate Frosting

This is a very rich and creamy frosting. Use it to frost the Double Chocolate Decadence Cake (see page 109) or any other 2-layer cake.

Preparation time: 10 minutes
Frosting time: 6 to 8 minutes

3 ounces dairy-free **unsweetened baking chocolate**
3¼ cups **powdered sugar**
¼ cup + 2 tablespoons dairy-free **margarine**, room temperature
⅓ cup dairy-free **vegetable shortening**
3 teaspoons water
1 teaspoon **pure vanilla extract**

Place chocolate in a small microwave-safe mixing bowl; melt in microwave oven following package directions.

While chocolate is melting, sift powdered sugar into a large mixing bowl. Add melted chocolate and remaining ingredients. Using an electric mixer set at medium speed beat until well mixed. Use frosting immediately to frost cake.

Makes about 2½ cups frosting,
enough to frost a 9-inch 2-layer cake.

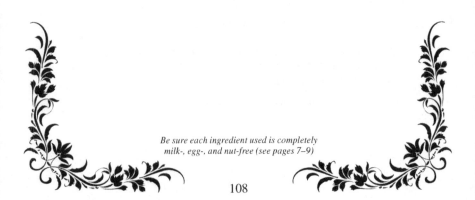

Be sure each ingredient used is completely milk-, egg-, and nut-free (see pages 7–9)

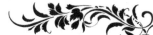

Double Chocolate Decadence Cake

Here's an extremely rich and chocolaty cake for all of you chocoholics! This is so rich that I usually serve it in pieces that are half the size of a "normal" slice of layer cake.

Preparation time: 15 minutes
Cooking time: 30 to 35 minutes

3 ounces dairy-free **unsweetened baking chocolate**
3 cups **all-purpose flour**
2 cups pure cane sugar
2 teaspoons **baking soda**
1½ cups **vanilla-flavored soy milk**
⅓ cup canola or **vegetable oil**
2 tablespoons canola or **vegetable oil**, 2 tablespoons water, and
    2 teaspoons **baking powder**, mixed together
2 cups dairy- and nut-free **semi-sweet chocolate chips**
Decadent Chocolate Frosting (see recipe on page 108)

Preheat oven to 375 degrees F. Using dairy-free **vegetable shortening**, grease and then flour two 9-inch round cake pans.

Place baking chocolate in a small microwave-safe bowl; melt in microwave oven following the package directions.

While chocolate is melting, sift flour, sugar, and baking soda into a large mixing bowl. Add melted chocolate, soy milk, oil, and oil/water/ baking powder mixture; mix well. Stir in chocolate chips.

Pour batter evenly into prepared cake pans. Bake for 30 to 35 minutes, or until a toothpick inserted into the center of the cake (but not into a melted chocolate chip) comes out clean. Cool in pans 10 minutes before turning out onto wire racks to cool completely. Use Decadent Chocolate Frosting to frost middle, top, and sides of layer cake.

Makes one 9-inch round 2-layer cake.

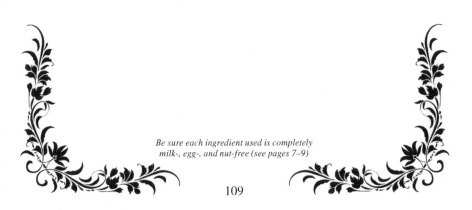

*Be sure each ingredient used is completely
milk-, egg-, and nut-free (see pages 7–9)*

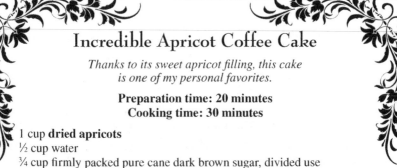

Incredible Apricot Coffee Cake

*Thanks to its sweet apricot filling, this cake
is one of my personal favorites.*

**Preparation time: 20 minutes
Cooking time: 30 minutes**

1 cup **dried apricots**
½ cup water
¾ cup firmly packed pure cane dark brown sugar, divided use
½ cup dairy-free **margarine**, room temperature
½ cup pure cane sugar
1⅔ cups **all-purpose flour**
¼ cup pineapple juice
1½ tablespoons canola or **vegetable oil**, 1½ tablespoons water,
    1 teaspoon **baking powder**, mixed together
1 teaspoon **baking soda**
1 teaspoon **pure vanilla extract**

Preheat oven to 400 degrees F. Using **vegetable oil**, generously grease
an 8-inch square baking pan.

To make apricot filling, cut the dried apricots into quarters. Place
apricot pieces and ½ cup water in a 1½- or 2-quart saucepan. Cover and
bring to a boil over high heat. Reduce heat to low and simmer, covered,
for about 7 minutes or until water is nearly absorbed and apricots are
tender. Remove from heat. Do not drain. Mash apricots slightly with the
back of a spoon. Stir in ½ cup brown sugar.

While filling is cooking, cream margarine, sugar, and ¼ cup brown
sugar together in a large mixing bowl. Add flour, pineapple juice,
oil/water/baking powder mixture, baking soda, and vanilla; mix well.
Note: Batter will be quite thick (like a cookie dough).

Place half of batter mixture into prepared pan; using wet hands, press
evenly into bottom of pan. Spread prepared filling evenly over batter.
Carefully top with remaining batter mixture, dropping batter by
the spoonful over the apricot filling. Don't worry if the filling is not
completely covered, as the batter will spread as it cooks. Bake for about
30 minutes, until top is golden brown and cake remains firm when the
pan is gently shaken from side to side. Cool in pan and then cut into
9 pieces before serving.

Makes 9 servings (about 2⅝ inches by 2⅝ inches each).

*Be sure each ingredient used is completely
milk-, egg-, and nut-free (see pages 7–9)*

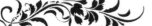

Lemon Cake with Blueberry Topping

This makes a very attractive cake, perfect for serving to company.

Cake preparation time: 12 minutes
Cooking time: 20 minutes
Topping time: 12 minutes

Cake

1½ cups **all-purpose flour**
⅔ cup pure cane sugar
½ cup water
⅓ cup canola or **vegetable oil**
1 tablespoon grated lemon peel
1 teaspoon **baking soda**
½ cup freshly squeezed lemon juice (about 3 lemons)
3 teaspoons **baking powder**

Topping

1¾ cups rinsed and drained frozen blueberries (measured after the
    berries are rinsed)
¼ cup pure cane sugar
2 tablespoons corn starch
1 tablespoon water

Preheat oven to 375 degrees F. Using dairy-free **vegetable shortening**,
grease and then flour a 9-inch round cake pan.

Place flour, ⅔ cup sugar, ½ cup water, oil, lemon peel, and baking
soda in a large mixing bowl. Place lemon juice and baking powder in
a small measuring cup; mix well. Add lemon juice mixture to rest of
cake ingredients in the mixing bowl; mix well. Pour batter evenly into
prepared pan. Bake for about 20 minutes, until a toothpick inserted into
the center of the cake comes out clean. Cool in pan for 10 minutes.

While cake cools, prepare blueberry topping. Place blueberries and
remaining ¼ cup sugar in a 1½- or 2-quart saucepan. Bring to a boil over
medium-high heat, stirring frequently. Place corn starch and water in a
small bowl or measuring cup; mix well and then add to boiling blueberry
mixture. Cook, stirring constantly, for about 30 seconds, until mixture
thickens. Remove from heat. Remove cake from pan and place on a
serving platter. Carefully spoon blueberry mixture evenly over top of
cake. Cool 20 minutes before serving.

Makes 6 to 8 servings.

*Be sure each ingredient used is completely
milk-, egg-, and nut-free (see pages 7–9)*

Marshmallow Frosting

This frosting, which is lighter than most egg-free frostings, can be a little tricky to work with. The keys are to work quickly and to use a margarine with a high fat content.

Preparation time: 8 to 10 minutes

2¾ cups **powdered sugar**
½ cup dairy-free **vegetable shortening**
¼ cup + 1 tablespoon dairy-free **margarine**, room temperature
2½ tablespoons **vanilla-flavored soy milk** or **rice milk**
2 cups dairy-, egg-, and nut-free **mini marshmallows**

Sift powdered sugar into a medium bowl; set aside. Measure shortening, margarine, and soy milk; set aside. Get out an electric mixer. You will not have time to measure things out once the marshmallows are melted.

Place marshmallows in a large microwave-safe bowl. Microwave on high for 30 seconds. Stir. If the marshmallows are not melted, continue to microwave in 15-second increments just until melted.

Working very quickly, add pre-measured powdered sugar, shortening, margarine, and soy or rice milk to the mixing bowl with the melted marshmallows. Using the electric mixer set at medium-high speed, beat until well mixed. Use immediately to frost cake; the frosting will "set" after it sits a little while.

Makes 2 cups.

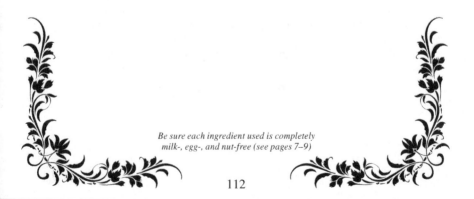

*Be sure each ingredient used is completely
milk-, egg-, and nut-free (see pages 7–9)*

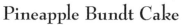

Pineapple Bundt Cake

A Bundt cake is a dessert cake that is baked in a Bundt pan or a round baking pan with a tube in the middle and fluted, decorated sides. Bundt cakes need little embellishment and, like this cake, are often served drizzled with a powdered sugar glaze.

Preparation time: 15 minutes
Cooking time: 50 minutes
Icing time: 5 minutes

1¼ cups **whole wheat flour**
1 cup **all-purpose flour**
½ cup pure cane sugar
½ cup firmly packed pure cane dark brown sugar
¼ cup **toasted wheat germ** (i.e., buy the variety that is called "toasted")
¼ cup canola or **vegetable oil**
2 tablespoons canola or **vegetable oil**, 2 tablespoons water, and 2 teaspoons **baking powder**, mixed together
2 teaspoons **baking soda**
2 teaspoons **pure vanilla extract**
1 (20 ounce) can **crushed pineapple in juice**, not drained
1 cup **powdered sugar**

Preheat oven to 350 degrees F. Using dairy-free **vegetable shortening**, grease and then flour a 7-cup Bundt pan.

Set aside 1 tablespoon plus 2 teaspoons of pineapple juice from the canned pineapple. Place all ingredients except reserved juice and powdered sugar in a large mixing bowl; mix well. Pour cake batter evenly into prepared Bundt pan. Bake for about 50 minutes, until the cake is golden brown and springy to the touch. Cool in pan for 10 minutes, and then turn out of pan onto a serving platter to cool completely.

Once cake has cooled, prepare icing. Sift powdered sugar into a medium mixing bowl. Add reserved pineapple juice; mix well. Spoon icing over top of cooled cake, so that some the icing slowly drips down the sides of the cake. Allow the icing to set for 30 minutes before serving cake.

Makes 12 servings.

Be sure each ingredient used is completely milk-, egg-, and nut-free (see pages 7–9)

Pretty in Pink Cherry Cupcakes

*When you want to make cupcakes instead of a layer cake,
these cherry-flavored treats can be just the thing.*

**Preparation time: 15 minutes
Cooking time: 25 minutes
Frosting time: 20 minutes**

Cake

1 (10 ounce) bottle **stem-free maraschino cherries** (about 30 cherries),
   not drained
3 cups **all-purpose flour**
1 cup pure cane sugar
½ cup canola or **vegetable oil**
⅓ cup **vanilla-flavored soy milk** or **rice milk**
3 tablespoons canola or **vegetable oil**, 3 tablespoons water, and
   2 teaspoons **baking powder**, mixed together
1 tablespoon **baking powder**

Frosting

2 cups + 1 tablespoon **powdered sugar**
¼ cup + 2 tablespoons dairy-free **margarine**, room temperature
¾ teaspoon **pure vanilla extract**
few drops **red food coloring**

Preheat oven to 350 degrees F. Line 18 regular cupcake/muffin cups
with paper liners.

Drain cherries, reserving liquid. Place 2 tablespoons of this liquid
aside for use in the frosting. Place cherries and ⅓ cup of the liquid in a
blender; process until cherries are very finely chopped. Place processed
cherry/liquid mixture and remaining cake ingredients in a large mixing
bowl; mix well with a wire whisk. Spoon batter into prepared cupcake
cups, filling each one ⅔ full. Bake for about 25 minutes, or until a
toothpick inserted into the center of a cupcake comes out clean. Cool in
pans for 5 minutes and then remove to wire racks to cool completely.

When cupcakes have cooled, make frosting. Sift powdered sugar into a
large mixing bowl. Add margarine, vanilla, red food coloring, and the
2 tablespoons of liquid that were set aside from the bottle of cherries.
Using an electric mixer set at medium-high speed beat until well mixed.
Be patient, as this may take a few minutes. Use frosting immediately to
generously frost the cupcakes.

Makes 18 cupcakes.

*Be sure each ingredient used is completely
milk-, egg-, and nut-free (see pages 7–9)*

Spice Cake

*This old-fashioned 2-layer spice cake looks and tastes
wonderful with a fluffy Marshmallow Frosting.*

**Preparation time: 10 minutes
Cooking time: 30 minutes**

3½ cups **all-purpose flour**
1⅓ cups pure cane sugar
1½ cups apple juice
1⅓ cups canola or **vegetable oil**
3 tablespoons **white distilled vinegar**
3 teaspoons **baking soda**
1 teaspoon ground cinnamon
1 teaspoon ground allspice
1 teaspoon ground cloves
Marshmallow Frosting (see recipe on page 112)

Preheat oven to 375 degrees F. Using dairy-free **vegetable shortening**,
grease and then flour two 9-inch round cake pans.

Place flour, sugar, apple juice, oil, vinegar, baking soda, cinnamon,
allspice, and cloves in a large mixing bowl; mix well with a wire whisk.
Pour batter evenly into prepared cake pans. Bake for 30 minutes or until
a toothpick inserted into the center of the cake comes out clean. Cool in
pans for 5 minutes, and then remove to wire racks to cool completely.
Use Marshmallow Frosting to frost middle, top, and sides of layer cake.

Makes one 9-inch round 2-layer cake.

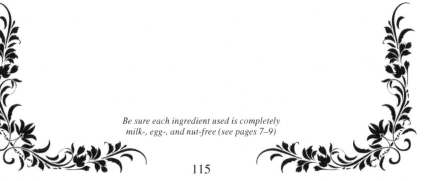

*Be sure each ingredient used is completely
milk-, egg-, and nut-free (see pages 7–9)*

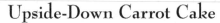

Upside-Down Carrot Cake

In this moist and dense twist on the traditional carrot cake I've substituted a sweet pineapple topping for the customary cream cheese frosting. If you're expecting a crowd you can double the recipe and bake it for 1 hour in a 9-inch by 13-inch cake pan.

Preparation time: 20 minutes
Cooking time: 55 to 60 minutes

3 tablespoons dairy-free **margarine**
1 (20 ounce) can **crushed pineapple packed in 100% pineapple juice**, not drained, divided use
⅓ cup + ¾ cup firmly packed pure cane dark brown sugar, divided use
½ cup honey
2 cups firmly packed, finely grated carrots (about ½ pound carrots)
1½ cups **whole wheat flour**
1 cup **all-purpose flour**
¼ cup canola or **vegetable oil**
2 teaspoons **pure vanilla extract**
2 teaspoons **baking soda**
1 teaspoon ground cinnamon
½ teaspoon ground allspice

Preheat oven to 350 degrees F.

Place margarine in an 8-inch square baking pan; place in oven until margarine melts, about 3 minutes. Meanwhile, drain pineapple, reserving juice. Place ½ cup crushed pineapple and ½ cup pineapple juice in a large mixing bowl; set aside. Discard remaining pineapple juice.

Sprinkle ⅓ cup brown sugar evenly over melted margarine in baking pan. Spoon remaining drained pineapple (i.e., all of the pineapple except for the ½ cup which is in the mixing bowl) evenly over brown sugar and margarine mixture in the pan; set aside.

Place honey in a small microwave-safe bowl or measuring cup. Microwave on high for about 30 seconds, until liquefied; stir. Add grated carrots, flours, remaining ¾ cup brown sugar, liquefied honey, oil, vanilla, baking soda, cinnamon, and allspice to pineapple in mixing bowl; mix well. Spoon batter evenly over the pineapple mixture in the pan. Bake for 55 to 60 minutes, until a toothpick inserted into the center of the cake comes out clean. Remove from oven and immediately invert onto a serving platter. If any of the topping sticks to the baking pan, quickly remove it with a rubber spatula, invert it onto the cake, and then smooth it into place. Cool completely before serving.

Makes 9 servings (approximately 2⅝ inches by 2⅝ inches each).

*Be sure each ingredient used is completely
milk-, egg-, and nut-free (see pages 7–9)*

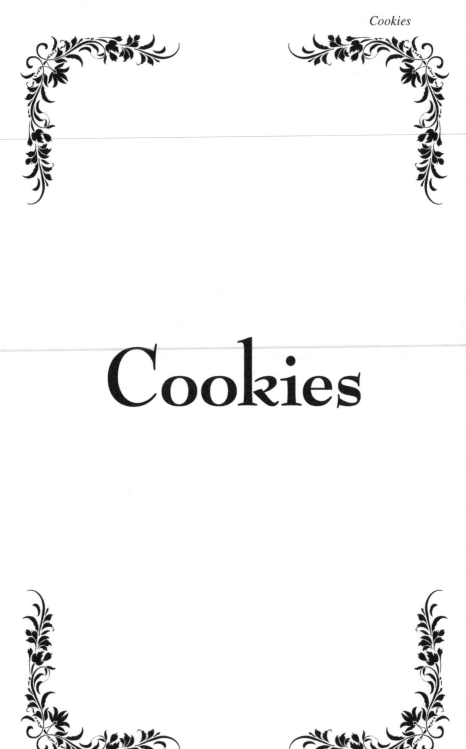

Cookies

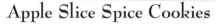

Apple Slice Spice Cookies

*Each of these hearty spice cookies are topped with a
slice of cinnamon- and sugar-coated apple. Yum!*

**Preparation time: 30 minutes
Cooking time: 15 minutes**

2½ tablespoons pure cane sugar
1¾ teaspoons ground cinnamon, divided use
2 medium-size Granny Smith apples
½ cup dairy-free **margarine**, room temperature
¾ cup firmly packed pure cane dark brown sugar
1½ cups **all-purpose flour**
2 tablespoons canola or **vegetable oil**, 2 tablespoons water, and
   1½ teaspoons **baking powder**, mixed together
1 tablespoon water
1 teaspoon **pure vanilla extract**
¼ teaspoon ground nutmeg
¼ teaspoon ground allspice

Preheat oven to 375 degrees F.

Place 2½ tablespoons sugar and ¾ teaspoon cinnamon in a medium
bowl; mix well. Peel and core apples. Cut each apple in half and then
slice each half into 12 thin slices. Add apple slices to cinnamon/sugar
mixture; toss gently to coat. Set aside.

Cream margarine and brown sugar together in a large mixing bowl. Add
flour, oil/water/baking powder mixture, 1 tablespoon water, vanilla,
remaining 1 teaspoon cinnamon, nutmeg, and allspice; mix well.

Spray cookie sheets with dairy-free **non-stick cooking spray**. Form
dough into 48 "logs," each approximately ½-inch wide by 1¾-inches
long. Place dough logs 2 inches apart on prepared cookie sheets. Press 1
prepared apple slice down onto each dough log, somewhat flattening the
cookie in the process. Bake for about 15 minutes, until edges of cookies
are set. Remove to wire racks to cool completely before serving.

Makes 48 (approximately 2-inch by 1½-inch) cookies.

Note: Cookies are best the day they are made. Avoiding stacking the cookies.

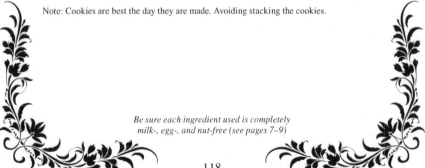

*Be sure each ingredient used is completely
milk-, egg-, and nut-free (see pages 7–9)*

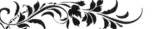
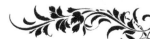

Apricot Oatmeal Chews

This is a delicious variation of the traditional oatmeal cookie.

Preparation time: 25 to 30 minutes
Cooking time: 12 minutes

1 cup quick-cooking oats
1 cup **dried apricots**
½ cup dairy-free **margarine**, room temperature
⅔ cup firmly packed pure cane dark brown sugar
⅓ cup pure cane sugar
1 cup **all-purpose flour**
2 tablespoons canola or **vegetable oil**, 2 tablespoons water, and
  1½ teaspoons **baking powder**, mixed together
1 teaspoon **pure vanilla extract**
¼ teaspoon ground cinnamon
¼ teaspoon ground nutmeg

Spread oats in a single layer on a shallow baking pan or rimmed cookie sheet. Turn on oven to 350 degrees F and place baking pan in oven for about 10 to 15 minutes or until oats are lightly toasted, stirring once during cooking time. Remove oats from baking pan and let cool in a separate bowl for 5 minutes.

While oats are toasting, chop dried apricots; set aside. Cream margarine and sugars together in a large mixing bowl. Add flour, oil/water/baking powder mixture, vanilla, cinnamon, and nutmeg; mix well. Add chopped apricots and toasted oats; mix well.

Form dough into 1¼-inch balls and place 2 inches apart on ungreased cookie sheets. Bake for about 12 minutes or until outer edges are set but cookies are still quite soft. Cool cookies on cookie sheets for 2 to 4 minutes and then remove to wire racks to cool completely.

Makes about 44 (2¼-inch diameter) cookies.

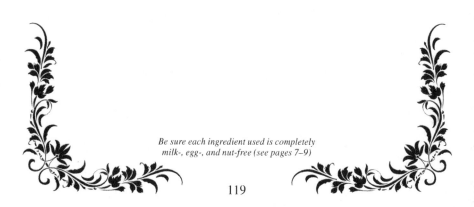

Be sure each ingredient used is completely
milk-, egg-, and nut-free (see pages 7–9)

Choco-Cherry Spritz Cookies

*These darling little cookies look like they
came straight from the bakery.*

**Preparation time: 20 to 25 minutes
Cooking time: 10 minutes
Icing time: 13 minutes**

1 cup dairy-free **margarine**, room temperature
2 cups **all-purpose flour**
1 cup **powdered sugar**
½ cup dairy-free unsweetened **cocoa powder**
1 (16 ounce) jar stem-free **maraschino cherries**, not drained
1 tablespoon canola or **vegetable oil**, 1 tablespoon water, and
    1 teaspoon **baking powder**, mixed together
1 teaspoon **pure vanilla extract**
1 cup dairy- and nut-free **semi-sweet chocolate chips**
1 teaspoon dairy-free **vegetable shortening**

Preheat oven to 375 degrees F.

Place margarine in a large mixing bowl; cream margarine using an
electric mixer set at high speed. Sift flour, powdered sugar, and cocoa
onto margarine. Add 2 tablespoons of liquid from the jar of maraschino
cherries, oil/water/baking powder mixture, and vanilla; mix well using
the electric mixer set at medium speed.

Fit cookie press with a cookie disk that will make a round cookie
without a hole in the center (avoid the "wreath" or "tree"-shaped disks).
Fill cookie press with cookie dough and form cookies 1 inch apart on
ungreased cookie sheets. Bake for about 10 minutes, until edges are set.
Cool on cookie sheets for 2 minutes and then remove to wire racks to
cool completely.

Drain cherries; discard liquid. Cut cherries in half; set aside. Place
chocolate chips and shortening in a small microwave-safe measuring
cup or bowl. Microwave on high for 45 seconds; stir. Continue to
microwave in 20-second increments until melted. Carefully spoon
some melted chocolate onto the middle of each cookie, and then press a
maraschino cherry half, cut side down, into the melted chocolate. Allow
chocolate to cool and harden before serving.

Makes about 55 to 60 small cookies (depending on size).

*Be sure each ingredient used is completely
milk-, egg-, and nut-free (see pages 7–9)*

Chocolate and Raisin Morsels

*This cookie's combination of melted chocolate chips
and sweet, chewy raisins is a real treat.*

Preparation time: 15 minutes
Cooking time: 8 to 10 minutes

½ cup dairy-free **margarine**, room temperature
⅓ cup firmly packed pure cane dark brown sugar
⅓ cup pure cane sugar
2 tablespoons canola or **vegetable oil**, 2 tablespoons water, and
   1 teaspoon **baking powder**, mixed together
1 teaspoon **pure vanilla extract**
1 cup **all-purpose flour**
1 cup **raisins**
1 cup dairy- and nut-free **semi-sweet chocolate chips**

Preheat oven to 350 degrees F.

Cream margarine and sugars together in a large mixing bowl. Add
oil/water/baking powder mixture and vanilla; mix well. Add flour;
mix well. Stir in raisins and chocolate chips.

Drop dough by rounded teaspoonfuls, 2 inches apart, onto ungreased
cookie sheets. Bake for about 8 to 10 minutes, until cookies are lightly
browned and outer edges are set. Cool on cookie sheets for 2 minutes
and then remove to wire racks to cool completely.

Makes about 56 bite-size (less than 2-inch diameter) cookies.

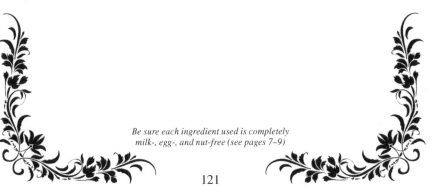

*Be sure each ingredient used is completely
milk-, egg-, and nut-free (see pages 7–9)*

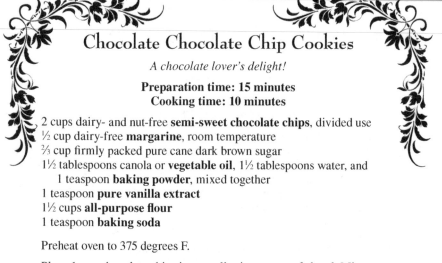

Chocolate Chocolate Chip Cookies

A chocolate lover's delight!

Preparation time: 15 minutes
Cooking time: 10 minutes

2 cups dairy- and nut-free **semi-sweet chocolate chips**, divided use
½ cup dairy-free **margarine**, room temperature
⅔ cup firmly packed pure cane dark brown sugar
1½ tablespoons canola or **vegetable oil**, 1½ tablespoons water, and
    1 teaspoon **baking powder**, mixed together
1 teaspoon **pure vanilla extract**
1½ cups **all-purpose flour**
1 teaspoon **baking soda**

Preheat oven to 375 degrees F.

Place 1 cup chocolate chips in a small microwave-safe bowl. Microwave
on high for 45 seconds; stir. Continue to microwave in 20-second
increments until melted. Let cool 1 minute.

Meanwhile, cream margarine and brown sugar together in a large
mixing bowl. Stir in the melted and cooled chocolate, oil/water/baking
powder mixture, and vanilla; mix well. Add flour and baking soda; mix
well. Stir in remaining 1 cup chocolate chips.

Form dough into 1-inch balls and place 2 inches apart on ungreased
cookie sheets. Bake for about 10 minutes, until the cookies look set but
are still somewhat soft to the touch. Cool on cookie sheets for 2 minutes
and then remove to wire racks to cool completely. Cookies will harden
as they cool.

Makes about 40 small cookies.

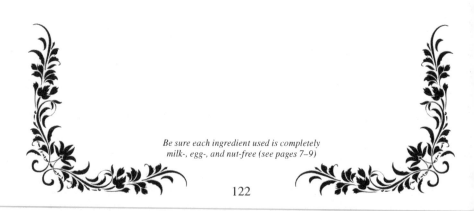

*Be sure each ingredient used is completely
milk-, egg-, and nut-free (see pages 7–9)*

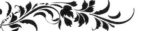

Cinnamon Sugar Cookies

*These buttery, cinnamon-flavored treats are crunchy
on the outside, soft and chewy on the inside.*

**Preparation time: 15 minutes
Cooking time: 10 minutes**

½ cup dairy-free **margarine**, room temperature
1 cup **powdered sugar**
1 cup **all-purpose flour**
1 teaspoon **baking powder**
1 tablespoon canola or **vegetable oil**, 1 tablespoon water, and
  1 teaspoon **baking powder**, mixed together
1 teaspoon **pure vanilla extract**
1¼ teaspoons ground cinnamon, divided use
1 tablespoon pure cane sugar

Preheat oven to 350 degrees F.

Place margarine in a large mixing bowl; sift in powdered sugar and
then cream margarine and sugar together. Sift in flour and 1 teaspoon
baking powder. Add oil/water/baking powder mixture, vanilla, and
1 teaspoon cinnamon; mix well.

Place 1 tablespoon sugar and remaining ¼ teaspoon cinnamon in a
small bowl; mix well. Form dough into 1-inch balls. Roll top of each
dough ball in the cinnamon/sugar mixture and then place the dough
balls, sugar side up, 2 inches apart on ungreased cookie sheets. Bake
for 10 to 11 minutes, until the outer edges of the cookies are starting to
set. The cookies will still be quite soft at this point; do not overcook as
they will harden as they cool. Cool on cookie sheets 2 minutes and then
remove to wire rack to cool completely.

Makes 26 (2-inch diameter) cookies.

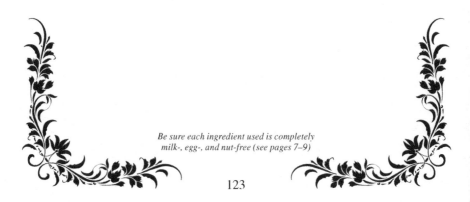

*Be sure each ingredient used is completely
milk-, egg-, and nut-free (see pages 7–9)*

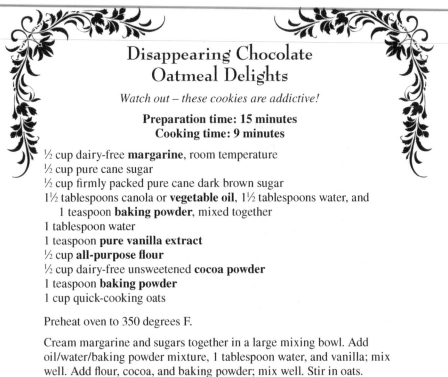

Disappearing Chocolate Oatmeal Delights

Watch out – these cookies are addictive!

Preparation time: 15 minutes
Cooking time: 9 minutes

½ cup dairy-free **margarine**, room temperature
½ cup pure cane sugar
½ cup firmly packed pure cane dark brown sugar
1½ tablespoons canola or **vegetable oil**, 1½ tablespoons water, and
    1 teaspoon **baking powder**, mixed together
1 tablespoon water
1 teaspoon **pure vanilla extract**
½ cup **all-purpose flour**
½ cup dairy-free unsweetened **cocoa powder**
1 teaspoon **baking powder**
1 cup quick-cooking oats

Preheat oven to 350 degrees F.

Cream margarine and sugars together in a large mixing bowl. Add oil/water/baking powder mixture, 1 tablespoon water, and vanilla; mix well. Add flour, cocoa, and baking powder; mix well. Stir in oats.

Drop dough by tablespoonfuls, 2 inches apart, onto ungreased cookie sheets. Bake for about 9 minutes, until the edges are firm but the rest of the cookie is still quite soft. Cool on cookie sheets 2 minutes before removing to wire racks to cool completely. Note: If after sitting for 2 minutes the cookies are still not firm enough to remove them from the cookie sheets, return them to the oven, cook for an additional 2 minutes, and then let sit for another 2 minutes before removing to wire racks to cool completely.

Makes 32 (2- to 2½-inch diameter) cookies.

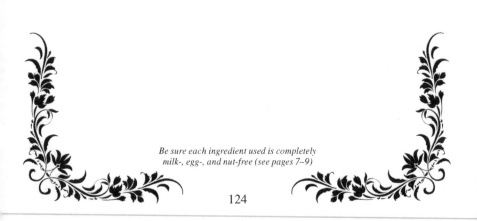

Be sure each ingredient used is completely milk-, egg-, and nut-free (see pages 7–9)

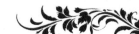

Double Chocolate Sweethearts

Looking for the perfect cookie to bake for your Valentine?
These very attractive heart-shaped treats are the answer!

Preparation time: 25 minutes
Cooking time: 10 minutes
Icing time: 13 minutes

1½ cups dairy- and nut-free **semi-sweet chocolate chips**, divided use
2¼ cups **all-purpose flour**
1 cup **powdered sugar**
1 teaspoon **baking powder**
1 cup dairy-free **margarine**, room temperature
1 tablespoon **white distilled vinegar**
1 tablespoon dairy-free **vegetable shortening**

Preheat oven to 350 degrees F.

Place ½ cup chocolate chips in a small microwave-safe bowl or measuring cup. Microwave on high for 30 seconds; stir. Continue to microwave in 15-second increments until melted.

Sift flour, powdered sugar, and baking powder into a large mixing bowl. Add margarine, vinegar, and melted chocolate. Using an electric mixer set at medium-high speed, beat until dough is well-mixed and forms a large clump. Be patient, as this will take a few minutes.

Roll out dough on a floured board to between ⅛- and ¼-inch thick. Cut out using a heart-shaped cookie cutter. Place cookies 1 inch apart on ungreased cookie sheets. Bake for about 9 to 10 minutes, just until edges are set. Note: Do not overcook, or cookies will be dry. Cool on cookie sheets for 2 minutes and then remove to wire racks to cool for 10 minutes.

To make icing, place shortening and remaining 1 cup chocolate chips in a small microwave-safe bowl or measuring cup. Microwave on high for 45 seconds; stir. Continue to microwave in 20-second increments until melted; stir. Using a frosting spatula, spread some icing on top of each cookie. Allow to cool completely before serving. If desired, place cookies in a single layer on cookie sheets and refrigerate until icing hardens.

Makes 50 (2½ inches wide) or
28 (3½ inches wide) heart-shaped cookies.

Be sure each ingredient used is completely
milk-, egg-, and nut-free (see pages 7–9)

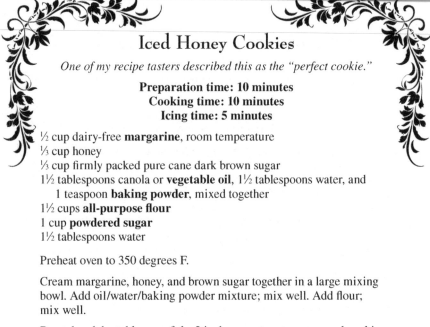

Iced Honey Cookies

One of my recipe tasters described this as the "perfect cookie."

Preparation time: 10 minutes
Cooking time: 10 minutes
Icing time: 5 minutes

½ cup dairy-free **margarine**, room temperature
⅓ cup honey
⅓ cup firmly packed pure cane dark brown sugar
1½ tablespoons canola or **vegetable oil**, 1½ tablespoons water, and
    1 teaspoon **baking powder**, mixed together
1½ cups **all-purpose flour**
1 cup **powdered sugar**
1½ tablespoons water

Preheat oven to 350 degrees F.

Cream margarine, honey, and brown sugar together in a large mixing bowl. Add oil/water/baking powder mixture; mix well. Add flour; mix well.

Drop dough by tablespoonfuls, 2 inches apart, onto ungreased cookie sheets. Bake for about 10 minutes, until bottoms of cookies are very lightly browned. Do not overcook, as cookies will harden as they cool. Cool on cookie sheets for 1 minute and then remove to wire racks to cool completely.

Once cookies have cooled, make icing. Sift powdered sugar into a medium mixing bowl. Stir in 1½ tablespoons water. Spoon some icing onto each cookie. Allow icing to harden before serving.

Makes 24 (about 2-inch diameter) cookies.

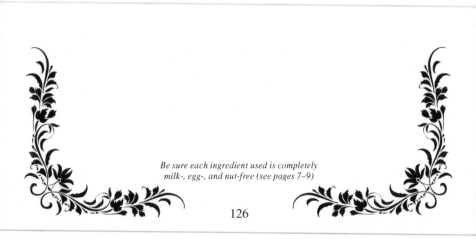

*Be sure each ingredient used is completely
milk-, egg-, and nut-free (see pages 7–9)*

Jack's Marbled Cookies

*Jack is a non-allergic member of my cookie-tasting team.
When his second grade class had a cookie exchange, he told
his father that he wanted to bring something that no one else
would bring, "like one of Linda's cookies." He chose these
because the marbled design makes them extra special!*

**Preparation time: 15 minutes
Cooking time: 12 minutes**

⅔ cup dairy- and nut-free **semi-sweet chocolate chips**
½ cup dairy-free **margarine**, room temperature
⅔ cup firmly packed pure cane dark brown sugar
¼ cup pure cane sugar
1½ cups **all-purpose flour**
2 tablespoons canola or **vegetable oil**, 2 tablespoons water, and
    2 teaspoons **baking powder**, mixed together
2 tablespoons water
2 teaspoons **pure vanilla extract**

Preheat oven to 375 degrees F.

Place chocolate chips in a small microwave-safe bowl or measuring
cup. Microwave on high for 45 seconds; stir. Continue to microwave in
20-second increments until melted. Set aside.

Cream margarine and sugars together in a large mixing bowl. Add
flour, oil/water/baking powder mixture, 2 tablespoons water, and
vanilla; mix well. Pour melted chocolate chips over cookie batter. Using
a rubber spatula, lightly fold melted chocolate into dough just until
chocolate is well-distributed and the dough has a marbled pattern. Do
not mix the chocolate completely into the dough.

Drop dough by heaping tablespoonfuls, 2 inches apart, onto ungreased
cookie sheets. Bake for about 12 minutes, until the outer ¼-inch of the
edges are set. Cool on cookie sheets for 2 minutes and then remove to
wire racks to cool completely. Note: If there isn't room in your oven
to bake the entire batch at once, be sure to cool the cookie sheets
completely before reusing them. These cookies tend to burn when
baked on preheated cookie sheets.

Makes about 23 (2¾-inch diameter) cookies.

*Be sure each ingredient used is completely
milk-, egg-, and nut-free (see pages 7–9)*

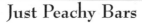

Just Peachy Bars

Between the jam and the pureed fruit, this thick, satisfying cookie bar has just the right amount of "peachiness."

Preparation time: 10 minutes
Cooking time: 30 minutes

1½ cups old-fashioned oats
1½ cups **all-purpose flour**
½ cup firmly packed pure cane dark brown sugar
½ teaspoon **baking soda**
¼ teaspoon ground allspice
½ cup dairy-free **margarine**, melted
1 (3.5 ounce) container **pureed peaches** (i.e., baby food)
⅔ cup **peach jam**

Preheat oven to 375 degrees F. Using dairy-free **vegetable shortening**, lightly grease an 8-inch square baking pan.

Place oats, flour, sugar, baking soda, and allspice in a large mixing bowl; mix well. Add melted margarine and pureed peaches; mix well.

Press half of oat mixture evenly onto bottom of prepared baking pan. Spread jam evenly over oat mixture. Break remaining oat mixture into small pieces, and use these pieces to evenly cover the layer of jam. Press down firmly. Bake for 30 minutes or until top is browned. Cool in pan 10 minutes and then cut into 16 squares.

Makes 16 bars (2 inches by 2 inches each).

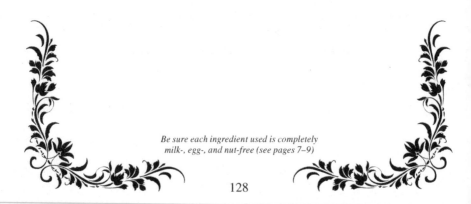

Be sure each ingredient used is completely milk-, egg-, and nut-free (see pages 7–9)

Molasses Chewies

*If you've got a craving for an old-fashioned molasses
cookie, this recipe is just what you're looking for!*

Preparation time: 15 minutes
Cooking time: 12 minutes

1 cup + 1 tablespoon pure cane sugar, divided use
1½ teaspoons ground cinnamon, divided use
½ cup dairy-free **margarine**, room temperature
2 cups **all-purpose flour**
¼ cup unsulfured **molasses**
1½ tablespoons canola or **vegetable oil**, 1½ tablespoons water, and
    1 teaspoon **baking powder**, mixed together
1 tablespoon water
2 teaspoons **baking soda**
1 teaspoon ground ginger

Preheat oven to 350 degrees F.

Place 1 tablespoon sugar and ½ teaspoon ground cinnamon in a small
bowl; mix well and then set aside.

Cream margarine and 1 cup sugar together in a large mixing bowl. Add
all remaining ingredients except the cinnamon/sugar mixture; mix well.

Form dough into 1-inch balls. Roll top of each dough ball in the
cinnamon/sugar mixture and then place the dough balls, sugar side up,
2 inches apart on ungreased cookie sheets. Bake for about 12 minutes,
until edges are set but middles of cookies are still somewhat soft. Cool
on cookie sheets 2 minutes and then remove to wire racks to cool
completely.

Makes 34 (about 2¼-inch diameter) cookies.

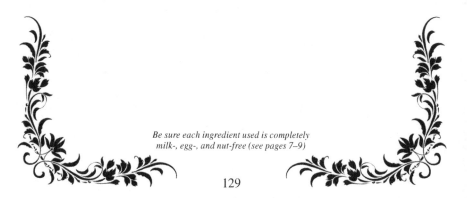

*Be sure each ingredient used is completely
milk-, egg-, and nut-free (see pages 7–9)*

Shortbread Thumbprint Cookies

*Try making half the batch with one variety of jam and half
with another, to see which flavor your family likes best.*

**Preparation time: 13 minutes
Cooking time: 15 minutes**

½ cup dairy-free **margarine**, room temperature
¼ cup pure cane sugar
1¼ cups **all-purpose flour**
2½ tablespoons **orange juice**
1 teaspoon **pure vanilla extract**
approximately ¼ cup **jam** or **jelly** of your choice

Preheat oven to 375 degrees F.

Cream margarine and sugar together in a large mixing bowl. Add flour,
orange juice, and vanilla; mix well.

Roll dough into 1-inch balls and place 2 inches apart on ungreased cookie
sheets. Use your thumb to make a deep indentation in the center of
each cookie (note: this will also somewhat flatten the cookie). Fill each
indentation with jam. Bake about 15 minutes, until edges are lightly
browned. Remove to wire racks to cool completely before serving.

Makes 20 (2-inch diameter) cookies.

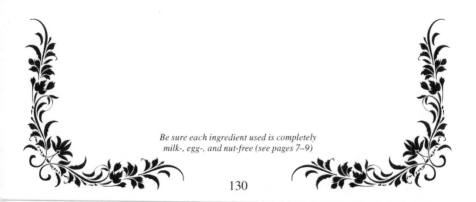

*Be sure each ingredient used is completely
milk-, egg-, and nut-free (see pages 7–9)*

Slice and Bake Cookies

To speed things up for this version of old-fashioned "refrigerator cookies," I place the dough in the freezer instead of the refrigerator. Of course, if you double the recipe and leave half the dough in the freezer you'll be ready to whip up a batch of fresh-baked cookies on a moment's notice some other day.

Dough preparation time: 8 minutes
Freezing time: 1 hour
Slice and decorate time: 4 minutes
Cooking time: 10 minutes

½ cup dairy-free **margarine**, room temperature
⅓ cup pure cane sugar
¼ cup firmly packed pure cane dark brown sugar
1½ cups **all-purpose flour**
1½ tablespoons canola or **vegetable oil**, 1½ tablespoons water, and
  1 teaspoon **baking powder**, mixed together
2 tablespoons **vanilla-flavored soy milk** or **rice milk**
Dairy-, egg-, and nut-free **colorful sprinkles**

Cream margarine and sugars together in a large mixing bowl. Add flour, oil/water/baking powder mixture, and soy or rice milk; mix well. Form dough into a 10-inch-long by 2-inch-diameter "log." Wrap log in plastic wrap and place in freezer for 1 hour. Note: If you will be leaving the dough in the freezer until another day, place the wrapped dough log in a freezer-proof plastic bag.

Preheat oven to 375 degrees F. Slice dough into ¼-inch slices and place 2 inches apart on ungreased cookie sheets. Decorate with colorful sprinkles. Bake for about 10 minutes, until edges barely begin to brown. Cool on cookie sheets for 1 minute and then remove to wire racks to cool completely.

Makes 26 (approximately 2-inch diameter) cookies.

Variation:

Chocolate Refrigerator Cookies

Follow recipe as above, except:
* Decrease **flour** to 1¼ cups
* Add ½ cup dairy-free unsweetened **cocoa powder**
* Increase **soy** or **rice milk** to 3 tablespoons; if desired use **chocolate-flavored soy** or **rice milk**

Be sure each ingredient used is completely milk-, egg-, and nut-free (see pages 7–9)

Two-Tones

*These cookies have a light-colored circular center
surrounded by a ring of chocolate.*

Preparation time: 15 minutes
Freezing time: 30 minutes
Cooking time: 14 minutes

½ cup dairy-free **margarine**, room temperature
⅓ cup + 1 tablespoon firmly packed pure cane dark brown sugar
⅓ cup pure cane sugar
1½ cups **all-purpose flour**
1½ tablespoons canola or **vegetable oil**, 1½ tablespoons water, and
    1 teaspoon **baking powder**, mixed together
1 tablespoon water
1 teaspoon **baking powder**
1 teaspoon **pure vanilla extract**
¼ cup dairy-free unsweetened **cocoa powder**
1 tablespoon honey

Cream margarine and sugars together in a large mixing bowl. Add
flour, oil/water/baking powder mixture, 1 tablespoon water, 1 teaspoon
baking powder, and vanilla; mix well.

Remove ¾ cup of dough from bowl. Form this dough into a 10-inch-
long "log." Set aside.

Sift cocoa into remaining dough. Add honey; mix well. Form this
chocolate dough into a ball. Place on an unfloured board and gently roll
out into a 10-inch by 4-inch rectangle. Place the white dough log onto
the chocolate rectangle. Carefully wrap the chocolate dough around
the white dough log; pinch edges to seal. Wrap two-tone dough log in
plastic wrap and place in freezer for 30 minutes.

Heat oven to 350 degrees F.

Remove dough from freezer; slice into ¼-inch-thick slices (note:
the slices tend to come out as ovals rather than the circles you might
expect). Place slices 2 inches apart on ungreased cookie sheet. Bake
for about 14 minutes, until the chocolate portion sets and becomes
somewhat firm to the touch. Remove to wire racks to cool.

Makes 32 cookies.

*Be sure each ingredient used is completely
milk-, egg-, and nut-free (see pages 7–9)*

Muffins, Quick Breads, & Breakfast Foods

Babke

My thanks go out to my dear friend Heidi for introducing
me to this delicious treat, which I would describe as being
somewhere between a coffee cake and a sweet bread.

Preparation time: 15 minutes
Cooking time: 1 hour

1 cup + 2 tablespoons pure cane sugar, divided use
1 teaspoon ground cinnamon
3 cups **all-purpose flour**
1¼ cups **vanilla-flavored soy milk**
¼ cup dairy-free **margarine**, melted
3 teaspoons **baking powder**
3 tablespoons canola or **vegetable oil**, 3 tablespoons water, and
 2 teaspoons **baking powder**, mixed together
1 teaspoon **pure vanilla extract**
½ cup **golden raisins** (optional)
1 tablespoon dairy-free **margarine**, cut up into small pieces

Preheat oven to 350 degrees F. Grease a 9-inch loaf pan with canola or
vegetable oil.

Place 2 tablespoons sugar and ground cinnamon in a small bowl; mix
well and then set aside.

Place flour, remaining 1 cup sugar, soy milk, melted margarine,
3 teaspoons baking powder, oil/water/baking powder mixture, and
vanilla in a large mixing bowl. Mix well with a wire whisk.

Spoon half of batter into prepared baking pan. Sprinkle with half of
cinnamon/sugar mixture, and then (if desired) sprinkle with raisins.
Carefully spoon remaining batter evenly over the cinnamon/sugar and
raisins. Sprinkle with remaining cinnamon/sugar mixture and then dot
with the cut-up pieces of margarine.

Bake for 1 hour, or until the top is golden brown and a toothpick
inserted into the center of the loaf comes out clean. Cool in pan
for 10 minutes, and then turn out onto wire rack. Cool for at least
30 minutes. Serve either warm or at room temperature.

Makes one 9-inch loaf.

Be sure each ingredient used is completely
milk-, egg-, and nut-free (see pages 7–9)

Banana Bread

When life gives you lemons, make lemonade. But when you're facing an oversupply of overripe bananas, this recipe is for you!

Preparation time: 12 to 15 minutes
Cooking time: 1 hour

3 medium-size bananas, either ripe or overripe
2 cups **all-purpose flour**
¾ cup pure cane sugar
¾ cup **apple sauce**
⅓ cup canola or **vegetable oil**
2 tablespoons canola or **vegetable oil**, 2 tablespoons water, and
    2 teaspoons **baking powder**, mixed together
1¼ teaspoons **baking soda**
¼ teaspoon ground nutmeg
⅛ teaspoon cloves

Preheat oven to 400 degrees F. Using dairy-free **vegetable shortening**, grease and then flour a 9-inch loaf pan.

Place bananas in a large mixing bowl; mash with a wooden spoon or potato masher, and then measure to ensure that you have about 1⅓ cups mashed banana.

Add remaining ingredients to bananas in mixing bowl; mix well using an electric mixer set at medium speed.

Pour batter into prepared loaf pan. Bake for 1 hour, or until a toothpick inserted into the center of the loaf comes out clean. Cool in pan for 10 minutes, and then remove from pan to wire rack to cool completely.

Makes one 9-inch loaf.

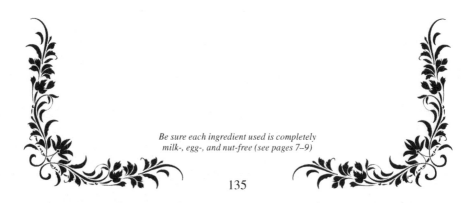

Be sure each ingredient used is completely milk-, egg-, and nut-free (see pages 7–9)

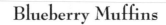

Blueberry Muffins

Good old-fashioned blueberry muffins – a perennial favorite!

Preparation time: 13 minutes
Cooking time: 25 minutes

2 cups **all-purpose flour**
¾ cup pure cane sugar
¾ cup **vanilla-flavored soy milk**
¼ cup dairy-free **margarine**, melted
1½ tablespoons canola or **vegetable oil**, 1½ tablespoons water, and
    1½ teaspoons **baking powder**, mixed together
2 tablespoons lemon juice (either freshly squeezed or bottled)
2 teaspoons **baking soda**
1½ cups unsweetened frozen blueberries, thawed and drained

Preheat oven to 375 degrees F. Line 11 regular muffin cups with paper muffin liners.

Place all ingredients except blueberries in a large mixing bowl; mix well. Using a rubber spatula, gently fold in blueberries.

Spoon batter into prepared muffin cups, filling each one so that it is full. Bake for about 25 minutes, until the tops are lightly browned and a toothpick inserted into the center of a muffin comes out clean. Cool at least 10 minutes before serving.

Makes 11 muffins.

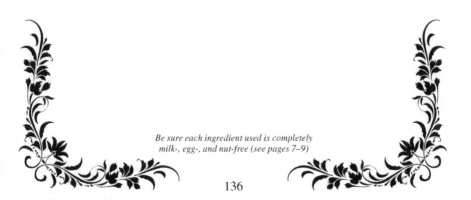

*Be sure each ingredient used is completely
milk-, egg-, and nut-free (see pages 7–9)*

Bran Muffins

A nice choice for breakfast or snacks.

Preparation time: 15 minutes
Cooking time: 25 minutes

2 cups **whole wheat flour**
1½ cups unprocessed **wheat bran**
⅔ cup firmly packed pure cane dark brown sugar
1 (6 ounce) can pineapple juice (¾ cup juice)
¾ cup boiling water
½ cup **applesauce**
¼ cup honey
¼ cup canola or **vegetable oil**
1½ tablespoons canola or **vegetable oil**, 1½ tablespoons water, and
   1 teaspoon **baking powder**, mixed together
2 teaspoons **baking soda**
1 teaspoon ground cinnamon
⅔ cup **golden raisins**

Preheat oven to 375 degrees F. Line 18 regular muffin cups with paper muffin liners.

Place all ingredients except raisins in a large mixing bowl; mix well. Stir in raisins. Spoon batter into prepared muffin cups, filling each one ¾ full. Bake for 25 minutes, or until a toothpick inserted into the center of a muffin comes out clean. Cool 10 minutes before serving.

Makes 18 muffins.

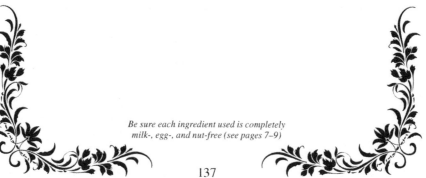

*Be sure each ingredient used is completely
milk-, egg-, and nut-free (see pages 7–9)*

Crumbcake Muffins

For me, these muffins are just another excuse to eat streusel topping!

Preparation time: 20 minutes
Cooking time: 25 minutes

Streusel Topping

¼ cup **all-purpose flour**
¼ cup firmly packed pure cane dark brown sugar
¼ cup pure cane sugar
½ teaspoon ground cinnamon
2 tablespoons dairy-free **margarine**, chilled

Muffins

2 cups **all-purpose** flour
1 cup apple juice (or one 6.75 ounce box of apple juice + 2 tablespoons
     water)
½ cup pure cane sugar
3 tablespoons canola or **vegetable oil**, 3 tablespoons water, and
     2 teaspoons **baking powder**, mixed together
2 tablespoons canola or **vegetable oil**
1 teaspoon **baking soda**
1 teaspoon **pure vanilla extract**
1 teaspoon ground cinnamon
1 teaspoon ground nutmeg

Preheat oven to 375 degrees F. Line 11 regular muffin cups with paper muffin liners.

To make streusel, place ¼ cup flour, ¼ cup brown sugar, ¼ cup sugar, and ½ teaspoon cinnamon in a medium mixing bowl; mix well. Using a pastry blender cut in the margarine until mixture resembles coarse crumbs; set aside.

Place remaining ingredients in a large mixing bowl; mix well.

Spoon batter into prepared muffin cups, filling each one ¾ full. Sprinkle a very generous spoonful of streusel topping over each muffin. Bake for 25 to 30 minutes, or until a toothpick inserted into the center of a muffin comes out clean. Cool at least 10 minutes before serving.

Makes 11 muffins.

Be sure each ingredient used is completely
milk-, egg-, and nut-free (see pages 7–9)

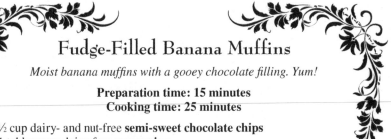

Fudge-Filled Banana Muffins

Moist banana muffins with a gooey chocolate filling. Yum!

Preparation time: 15 minutes
Cooking time: 25 minutes

½ cup dairy- and nut-free **semi-sweet chocolate chips**
1 tablespoon dairy-free **margarine**
3 medium-size ripe or overripe bananas
⅓ cup dairy-free **margarine**, melted
1½ tablespoons canola or **vegetable oil**, 1½ tablespoons water, and
    1 teaspoon **baking powder**, mixed together
1 teaspoon **pure vanilla extract**
1½ cups **all-purpose flour**
¾ cup pure cane sugar
1 teaspoon **baking soda**

Preheat oven to 375 degrees F. Line 11 regular muffin cups with paper muffin liners.

To make fudge filling, place chocolate chips and 1 tablespoon margarine in a small microwave-safe bowl. Microwave on high for 45 seconds; stir. Continue to microwave in 20-second increments until melted; stir until smooth and then set aside.

Place bananas in a large mixing bowl; mash with a wooden spoon or potato masher, and then measure to ensure that you have about 1⅓ cups mashed banana. Add ⅓ cup melted margarine, oil/water/baking powder mixture, and vanilla to the mashed bananas in the mixing bowl; mix well. Add flour, sugar, and baking soda; mix just until ingredients are combined.

Spoon batter into prepared muffin cups, filling each one ¼ full. Divide fudge filling between the 11 muffins, spooning about 2 teaspoons of filling onto each one. Carefully spoon remaining batter over chocolate, filling each muffin cup nearly full. Bake approximately 25 minutes, or until tops are browned. Cool 15 minutes before removing from muffin pan. Serve warm, while the fudge filling is melted. If fudge filling solidifies, briefly rewarm in a microwave oven.

Makes 11 muffins.

*Be sure each ingredient used is completely
milk-, egg-, and nut-free (see pages 7–9)*

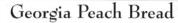

Georgia Peach Bread

Full of little pieces of chopped peaches, this bread makes a terrific snack or breakfast treat. Although all that fruit sometimes causes the slices to crumble a little, this peach bread is so good that you won't mind the mess.

Preparation time: 12 minutes
Cooking time: 1 hour

1 cup frozen peaches, thawed and drained
1¼ cups **whole wheat flour**
¾ cup **all-purpose flour**
¾ cup pure cane sugar
1 cup canned **peach nectar**
¼ cup canola or **vegetable oil**
2 tablespoons canola or **vegetable oil**, 2 tablespoons water, and
    2 teaspoons **baking powder**, mixed together
2 teaspoons **baking soda**
2 teaspoons **pure vanilla extract**
½ teaspoon ground allspice

Preheat oven to 375 degrees F. Using dairy-free **vegetable shortening**, grease and then flour a 9-inch loaf pan.

Finely chop peaches; set aside.

Place remaining ingredients in a large mixing bowl; mix just until ingredients are combined. Using a rubber spatula, fold in chopped peaches.

Pour batter into prepared loaf pan. Bake for about 1 hour, or until a toothpick inserted into the center of the loaf comes out clean. Cool in pan for 10 minutes. Remove to wire rack to cool completely before serving.

Makes one 9-inch loaf.

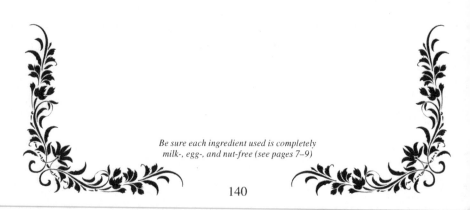

Be sure each ingredient used is completely milk-, egg-, and nut-free (see pages 7–9)

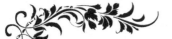
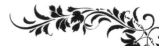

Granola

If you can't find a safe prepackaged granola, make your own!

Preparation time: 5 to 7 minutes
Cooking time: 15 minutes

3 tablespoons firmly packed pure cane dark brown sugar
3 tablespoons pure **maple syrup**
2 tablespoons honey
1 tablespoon canola or **vegetable oil**
1 teaspoon **pure vanilla extract**
¼ teaspoon ground cinnamon
¼ teaspoon ground nutmeg
2½ cups old-fashioned oats
½ cup **mixed dried fruit bits** (look for the type that includes raisins, apples, apricots, and peaches)

Preheat oven to 350 degrees F. Spray a rimmed cookie sheet with dairy-free **non-stick cooking spray**.

Place brown sugar, maple syrup, honey, oil, vanilla, cinnamon, and nutmeg in a 2-quart saucepan. Cook over low heat, stirring constantly, about 30 seconds, until sugar melts and sauce is well blended. Remove pan from heat. Stir in oats.

Spread mixture evenly on prepared cookie sheet. Bake for 10 minutes. Sprinkle dried fruit over granola mixture; stir and then spread mixture out evenly on the cookie sheet. Bake for an additional 5 minutes.

Remove granola from oven; stir. Cool on cookie sheet for 10 minutes, and then remove to a heat-proof serving bowl to cool completely.

Makes 3¾ cups.

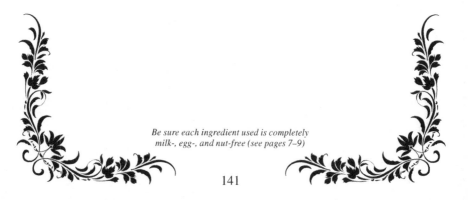

Be sure each ingredient used is completely
milk-, egg-, and nut-free (see pages 7–9)

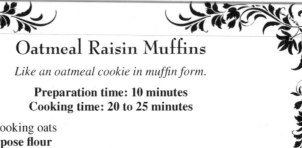

Oatmeal Raisin Muffins

Like an oatmeal cookie in muffin form.

Preparation time: 10 minutes
Cooking time: 20 to 25 minutes

1 cup quick-cooking oats
1 cup **all-purpose flour**
¾ cup apple juice
⅔ cup **raisins**
⅓ cup + 2 tablespoons firmly packed pure cane dark brown sugar
¼ cup dairy-free **margarine**, melted
3 tablespoons canola or **vegetable oil**, 3 tablespoons water, and
    2 teaspoons **baking powder**, mixed together
1 teaspoon **baking soda**
1 teaspoon ground cinnamon

Preheat oven to 400 degrees F. Line 9 regular muffin cups with paper muffin liners.

Place all ingredients in a large mixing bowl; mix well. Spoon batter into prepared muffin cups, filling each one nearly full. Bake for 20 to 25 minutes, or until the tops are golden brown and a toothpick inserted into the center of a muffin comes out clean. Cool 10 minutes before serving.

Makes 9 muffins.

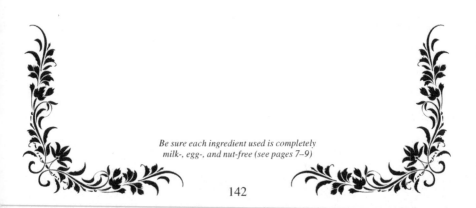

Be sure each ingredient used is completely milk-, egg-, and nut-free (see pages 7–9)

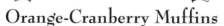

Orange-Cranberry Muffins

*These muffins are just right for rounding
out a breakfast or brunch menu.*

Preparation time: 13 minutes
Cooking time: 20 to 25 minutes

½ cup dairy-free **margarine**, room temperature
¾ cup pure cane sugar
2½ cups **all-purpose flour**
¾ cup water
¼ cup **orange juice**
3 tablespoons canola or **vegetable oil**, 3 tablespoons water, and
    2 teaspoons **baking powder**, mixed together
1 teaspoon **pure vanilla extract**
2 teaspoons **baking soda**
1 tablespoon freshly grated orange peel
½ cup **sweetened dried cranberries**

Preheat oven to 400 degrees F. Line 12 regular muffin cups with paper
muffin liners.

In a large mixing bowl, cream together margarine and sugar. Add flour,
water, orange juice, oil/water/baking powder mixture, vanilla, baking
soda, and grated orange peel; mix well. Stir in cranberries.

Spoon batter into prepared muffin cups, filling each one nearly full.
Bake for 20 to 25 minutes, until the tops are lightly browned and a
toothpick inserted into the center of a muffin comes out clean. Cool
10 minutes before serving.

Makes 12 muffins.

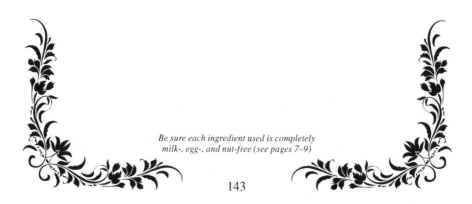

*Be sure each ingredient used is completely
milk-, egg-, and nut-free (see pages 7–9)*

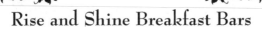

Rise and Shine Breakfast Bars

*These not-too-sweet breakfast bars have a wholesome
whole wheat taste that really grows on you.*

**Preparation time: 15 minutes
Cooking time: 30 to 35 minutes**

½ cup dairy-free **margarine**, room temperature
⅓ cup + 2 tablespoons firmly packed pure cane dark brown sugar
¼ cup honey
2 cups **whole wheat flour**
3 tablespoons canola or **vegetable oil**, 3 tablespoons water, and
   1½ teaspoons **baking powder**, mixed together
2 tablespoons apple juice
1 teaspoon **baking powder**
1 cup **jam** or **sugar-free fruit spread** (any flavor)

Preheat oven to 375 degrees F. Using canola or **vegetable oil**, grease an
8-inch square baking pan.

Cream margarine, brown sugar, and honey together in a large mixing
bowl. Add flour, oil/water/baking powder mixture, apple juice, and
1 teaspoon baking powder; mix well.

Press half of dough evenly onto bottom of prepared pan. Spread jam
evenly over dough. Break remaining dough up into small pieces and
drop evenly over jam. Bake for 30 to 35 minutes or until top is crunchy
and golden. Cool 10 minutes and then cut into 9 squares.

Makes 9 servings (approximately 2⅝ inches by 2⅝ inches each).

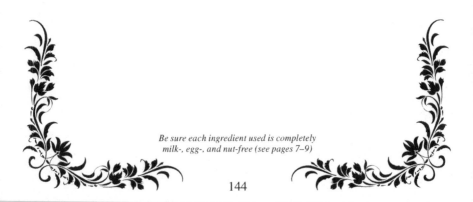

*Be sure each ingredient used is completely
milk-, egg-, and nut-free (see pages 7–9)*

Wholesome Snack Muffins

*Inspired by a giant zucchini that grew in my garden,
these relatively healthy treats resemble a cross between
zucchini bread, carrot cake, and bran muffins.*

Preparation time: 15 minutes
Cooking time: 35 minutes

¾ pound zucchini
¼ pound carrots
2 cups **whole wheat flour**
1 cup unprocessed **wheat bran**
1 cup **orange juice**
½ cup pure cane sugar
½ cup firmly packed pure cane dark brown sugar
3 tablespoons canola or **vegetable oil**, 3 tablespoons water, and
    2 teaspoons **baking powder**, mixed together
3 tablespoons canola or **vegetable oil** (in addition to oil listed above)
1 teaspoon **baking soda**
1 teaspoon ground cinnamon
½ teaspoon ground allspice

Preheat oven to 375 degrees F. Line 16 regular muffin cups with paper
muffin liners.

Trim ends off zucchini. Using a food processor that has been fitted
with the grating disk, grate zucchini. Measure grated zucchini to
ensure that you have 2 cups; set aside. Grate and then measure carrots;
you should have 1 cup. Replace grating disk with metal blade and
place the grated vegetables back into the bowl of the food processor;
process until vegetables are very finely chopped (yes, I am asking you
to chop the vegetables that you just grated – the consistency comes out
better this way).

Place all ingredients (including prepared zucchini and carrots) in a
large mixing bowl; mix well.

Spoon batter into prepared muffin cups, filling each one until it is full.
Bake for about 35 minutes, until a toothpick inserted into the center of
a muffin comes out clean. Cool 10 to 15 minutes before serving.

Makes 16 muffins.

*Be sure each ingredient used is completely
milk-, egg-, and nut-free (see pages 7–9)*

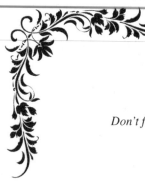

Menu Ideas

Don't forget to double-check the ingredients
on all purchased items!

PARTIES

Fourth of July Barbecue

Avocado Dip (page 99) served with Tortilla Chips
Platter of Raw Fresh Vegetables (such as carrot and celery sticks, etc.)
Linda's Signature Grilled Chicken (page 49)
Grilled Zucchini Ribbons (page 90)
Tabbouleh Salad with Sun-Dried Tomatoes (page 28)
Fruited Pasta Salad (page 63)
Double Chocolate Decadence Cake (page 109)
Cinnamon Sugar Cookies (page 123)

Mother's Day Luncheon

Sun-Dried Tomato Spread (page 103) served with Water Crackers
Critics' Choice Chicken Salad (page 20)
Fresh Strawberries
Bran Muffins (page 137)

DINNER FOR GUESTS

Company's Coming #1

Jason's Four-Star Brisket (page 33)
Steamed White Rice
Steamed Fresh Green Beans
Iced Honey Cookies (page 126)

Company's Coming #2

Spinach and Apple Salad (page 27)
Chicken Marsala (page 43)
Rice Pilaf (page 82)
Italian Vegetable Sauté (page 91)
Lemon Cake with Blueberry Topping (page 111)

Be sure each ingredient used is completely
milk-, egg-, and nut-free (see pages 7–9)

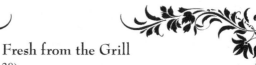

Fresh from the Grill

Steak on a Stick (page 38)
Grilled Potatoes (page 71)
Grated Zucchini Sauté (page 88)
Just Peachy Bars (page 128)

Lots of Fresh Herbs

California Sunburst Salad (page 18)
Four Ingredient Chicken (page 45)
Macaroni Verde (page 65)
Lemon-Basil Cauliflower (page 93)
Pineapple Bundt Cake (page 113)

FAMILY MEALS

Diner Special

Mom's Meat Loaf (page 34)
Mashed Potatoes (page 72)
Fresh Steamed Vegetables
Fresh Peach Crumble (page 102)

Fish Dinner

Fast and Easy Red Snapper (page 58)
Orange Vegetables (page 94)
Molasses Chewies (page 129)

Kid-Pleasing #1

Sloppy Joe Wraps (page 36)
Melon Balls
Chocolate Chocolate Chip Cookies (page 122)

Kid-Pleasing #2

Jammin' Chicken (page 48) or Fried Chicken Tenders (page 46)
Candied Carrots (page 86)
Baked Potatoes

Soups On

Slow Cooker Chicken and Vegetable Soup (page 25)
French Bread or Baguette

*Be sure each ingredient used is completely
milk-, egg-, and nut-free (see pages 7–9)*

Stir-Fry Dinner
Stir-Fried Beef with Sugar Snap Peas (page 40)
Steamed White Rice
Disappearing Chocolate Oatmeal Delights (page 124)

Sunday Supper
Best-Loved Roasted Chicken Dinner (page 42)
Apple Sauce
Cherry Streusel Cake (page 106)

30-Minute Pasta Dinner
Farmer's Market Pasta (page 62)
Fresh Watermelon

LUNCH
Cold Wraps
Veggie Wraps (page 104)
Potato Chips

Hot Wraps
Plum Sauced Chicken in Tortillas (page 51)
Fresh Strawberries

No Time to Cook Soup and Salad
Seven Minute Soup (page 24)
Fresh Green Salad with Vinaigrette

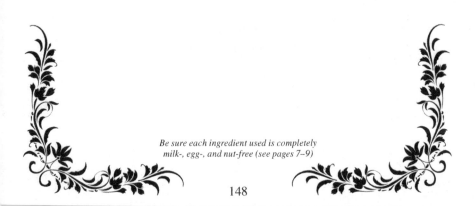

*Be sure each ingredient used is completely
milk-, egg-, and nut-free (see pages 7–9)*

Glossary

Bake: To cook, covered or uncovered, by dry heat (usually in an oven). When applied to meats, poultry, or vegetables cooked uncovered, the process is called roasting.

Baste: To brush or spoon a liquid (such as pan drippings, melted fat, sauce, or other seasoned liquid) over food, in order to add flavor and increase moisture.

Beat: To stir or mix rapidly in a quick, even, circular motion, in order to make a mixture smooth, lighter, or fluffier. When using a spoon or wire whisk, lift mixture up and over with each stroke.

Blend: To thoroughly combine two or more ingredients until smooth and uniform in texture, color, and flavor.

Broil: To cook by direct heat in the broiler of an electric or gas range.

Chop: To cut food into small pieces.

Coat: To cover a food with a surface layer of another ingredient, such as flour, by sprinkling, dipping, or rolling.

Combine: To stir two or more ingredients together until blended.

Core: To remove the center of a fruit or vegetable.

Cream: To beat with a spoon or an electric mixer until soft, smooth, and fluffy, as in blending margarine and sugar.

Cut in: To distribute solid fat, such as margarine, into dry ingredients with a pastry blender until particles are the desired size.

Fold in: To incorporate a delicate substance into another substance. A rubber spatula is used to gently bring part of the mixture from the bottom of the bowl to the top. The process is repeated, while slowly rotating the bowl, until the ingredients are blended.

Grease and flour pan: A process for coating a baking pan in order to prevent the finished baked good from sticking to the pan. Using a folded napkin or paper towel, coat the entire inside surface of the pan with the specified "grease" (such as vegetable shortening). Then place a spoonful of flour in the baking pan. Shake the pan to coat

Be sure each ingredient used is completely milk-, egg-, and nut-free (see pages 7–9)

the entire inside surface with a fine layer of flour, then shake out any excess flour from the pan.

Marinate: To soak food in a (usually acidic) liquid in order to tenderize the food or to enhance its flavor.

Mince: To chop or cut food into very small pieces.

Mix: To stir or beat two or more ingredients together until they are thoroughly combined and form a uniform mixture.

Preheat: To heat oven to desired temperature before beginning to cook.

Puree: To mash foods until perfectly smooth, usually by whirling in a blender or food processor.

Roast: To cook uncovered meats, poultry, or vegetables by dry heat (usually in an oven).

Sauté: To cook food in a pan in a small quantity of hot oil, usually stirring frequently during the cooking process.

Seed: To remove the seeds from fruits or vegetables.

Shred: To cut or grate food into thin, irregular strips.

Sift: To pass dry ingredients, such as flour or powdered sugar, through a sifter or sieve to remove lumps and aerate the ingredients.

Simmer: To cook in liquid just below the boiling point. The surface of the liquid should be barely moving, broken from time to time by slowly rising bubbles.

Skillet: A long-handled, round pan with a flat bottom and sloping sides that is used for cooking foods.

Steam: To cook in water vapors, on a rack or in a steam basket above boiling water, in a covered pot or pan.

Stir-fry: A method of quickly cooking small pieces of food in a small amount of hot oil in a wok or skillet over high heat, stirring constantly.

Toss: To combine ingredients with a lifting motion.

To taste: To add an ingredient to a recipe in a quantity based on the personal preference of the cook.

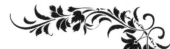

Food Allergy Resources

Please visit my website, *www.FoodAllergyBooks.com*, for an extensive list of current food allergy resources, including:

- Support groups
- General food allergy information
- Allergen-free foods
- Products for carrying allergy medications
- Clothing, buttons, and stickers
- Other useful food allergy products
- Blogs and e-newsletters
- Patient organizations
- Medical organizations
- Free downloadable food allergy resources
  - Pamphlets and posters
  - Sample forms and letters
  - Chef's cards
  - School and camp information

Measurement Equivalents

3 teaspoons	=	1 tablespoon
½ tablespoon	=	1½ teaspoons
4 tablespoons	=	¼ cup
5 tablespoons + 1 teaspoon	=	⅓ cup
8 tablespoons	=	½ cup
10 tablespoons + 2 teaspoons	=	⅔ cup
12 tablespoons	=	¾ cup
16 tablespoons	=	1 cup
¼ cup + 2 tablespoons	=	⅜ cup
½ cup + 2 tablespoons	=	⅝ cup
¾ cup + 2 tablespoons	=	⅞ cup
1 cup	=	8 fluid ounces
2 cups	=	1 pint
2 pints	=	1 quart
4 quarts	=	1 gallon

Index

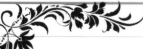

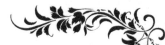

Contact the Author

Dear Reader,

I sincerely hope that this book helps make it easy for you to prepare delicious foods that your entire family can enjoy.

I would love to hear from you! Please send me your comments, questions, and feedback on *What Else is to Eat? The Dairy-, Egg-, and Nut-Free Food Allergy Cookbook.*

I can be reached via email at:
    LindaCoss@FoodAllergyBooks.com

Or via snail-mail at:
    Linda Coss
    Plumtree Press
    P.O. Box 1313, Dept. B3
    Lake Forest, CA 92609-1313

Thank you!

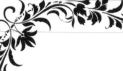

Order Form

Also available online at *www.FoodAllergyBooks.com*

For mail orders, please **photocopy** this form, fill it out, and mail it with payment (in U.S. dollars only) to:

Plumtree Press
P.O. Box 1313, Dept. B3
Lake Forest, CA 92609-1313

Quantity	Book Title	Each	Total
	What's to Eat? Cookbook	$16.95	
	What Else is to Eat? Cookbook	$16.95	
	How to Manage Your Child's Life-Threatening Food Allergies	$16.95	
	SUBTOTAL		
	Shipping and Handling Priority Mail to U.S. addresses: $6 for 1 or 2 books, $10 for 3 books Canadian orders: $9 for 1 or 2 books, $13 for 3 books		
	TOTAL		

Note: Prices and availability subject to change without notice.

Name: _____

Address: _____

_____

E-mail (optional): _____

2008